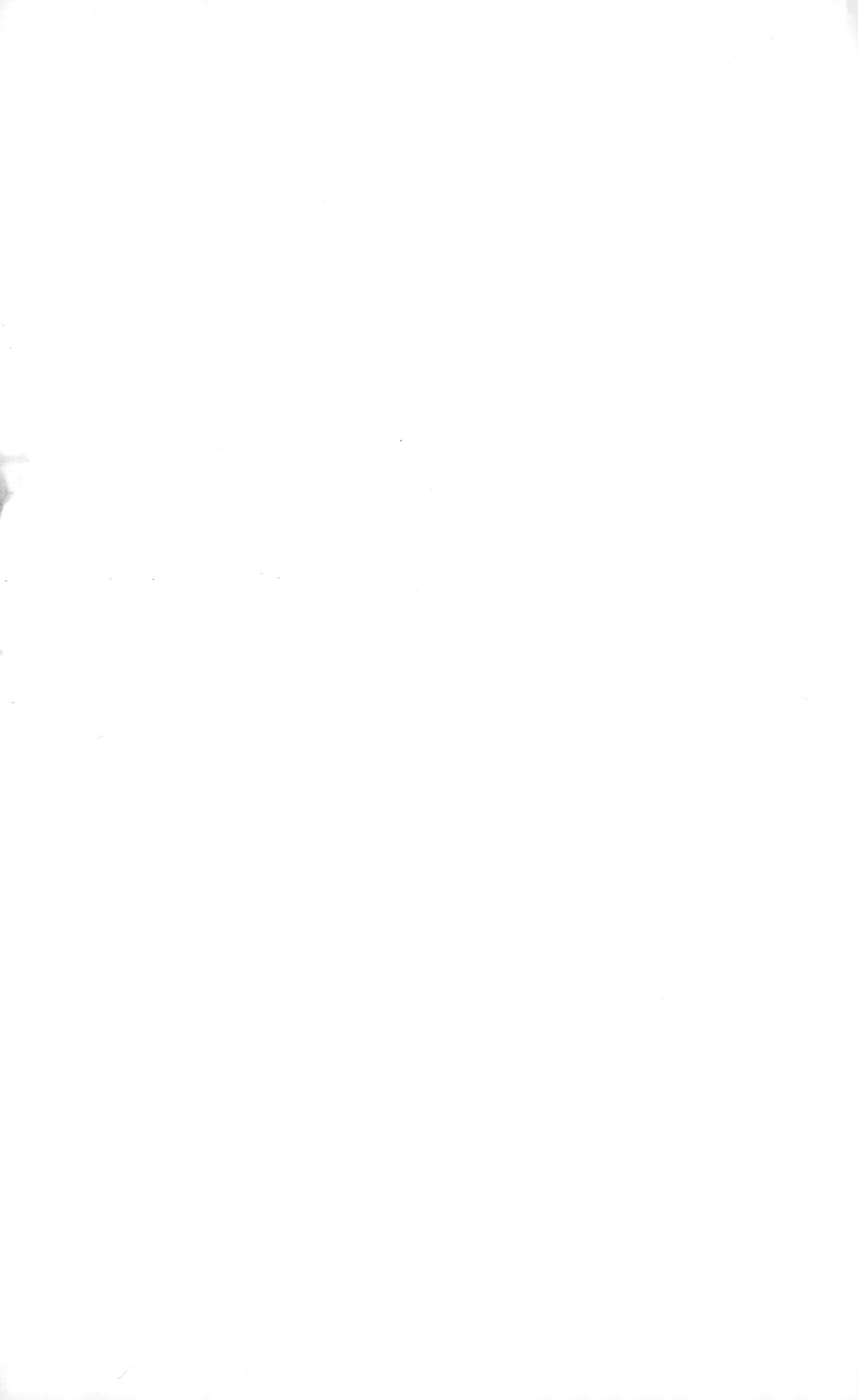

Hands-on Experiments in Agronomy & Crop Physiology

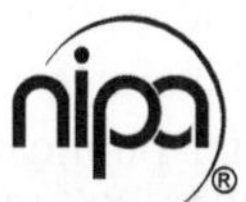

NIPA® GENX ELECTRONIC RESOURCES & SOLUTIONS P. LTD.
New Delhi-110 034

About the Author

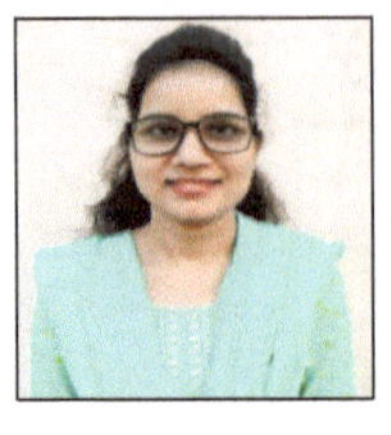

Dr. Kavita Solanki has completed her B.Sc. (Ag.) and M.Sc. (Ag.) in Agronomy from Rajmata Vijayaraje Scindia Krishi Vishwavidyalaya, Gwalior (Madhya Pradesh) in 2018 and 2020 respectively. She received her Ph. D in Agronomy from Dr. Rajendra Prasad Central Agricultural University, Pusa (Bihar) in 2024. She has cleared ASRB-NET in 2021. Her publication portfolio includes 8 research papers, 3 reviews, 13 book chapters, 2 authored books, and 20 popular articles and participated in conferences, seminars, trainings and workshops..

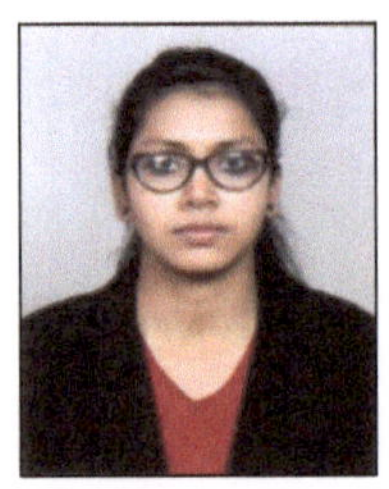

Dr. Jyostnarani Pradhan is currently working as Assistant Professor in the Department of Botany, Plant Physiology and Biochemistry, College of Basic Sciences and Humanities, Dr. Rajendra Prasad Central Agriculture University, Pusa, Samastipur, Bihar. She pursued her Ph.D. degree in the Department of Plant Physiology, Institute of Agricultural Sciences, Banaras Hindu University. She did her bachelor and master degree from Odisha University of Agriculture and Technology, Bhubaneswar. She worked under many national and international scientists during her working period at CSISA project funded by IRRI and attended training programme at IRRI head quarter, Philippines. She has been awarded with award of excellence and gold medal for her performance during masters. Her several research papers and articles have been published in national and international journals.

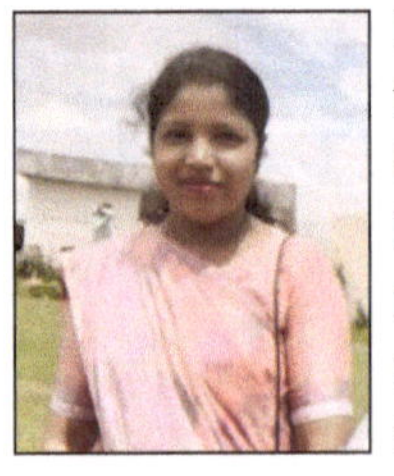

Dr. Hemlata Singh is an Assistant Professor of Biochemistry at the Department of Botany, Plant Physiology, and Biochemistry, CBSH, Dr. Rajendra Prasad Central Agricultural University, Pusa, Bihar. With expertise in nutritional biochemistry, metabolomics, and post-harvest physiology, she has extensive research experience in studying biochemical changes under stress and improving crop shelf life. Previously, Dr. Singh worked as a Consultant Scientist at Monsanto India Ltd., contributing to Vegetable Quality Analytics. She has supervised 1 M.Sc. student as the major advisor and co-advised 15 M.Sc. and 1 Ph.D. students. Currently, she leads an institute-funded project as PI, collaborates on externally funded projects, and contributes to AICRP initiatives. Her publication portfolio includes 10 research papers, 5 reviews, 8 book chapters, 1 edited book, and 10 popular articles, with 115 citations, an h-index of 7, and an i10-index of 6, showcasing her significant contributions to plant biochemistry research.

Hands-on Experiments in Agronomy & Crop Physiology

Kavita Solanki
Assistant Professor
Sanjeev Agrawal Global Educational (SAGE) University
Bhopal, Madhya Pradesh

Jyostnarani Pradhan
Assistant Professor
Department of Botany, Plant Physiology and Biochemistry
College of Basic Sciences and Humanities
Dr. Rajendra Prasad Central Agriculture University
Pusa, Samastipur, Bihar

Hemlata Singh
Assistant Professor
Department of Biochemistry
College of Basic Sciences & Humanities, Dr. Rajendra Prasad Central
Agricultuiral University, Pusa, Samastipur, Bihar

NIPA® GENX ELECTRONIC RESOURCES & SOLUTIONS P. LTD.
New Delhi-110 034

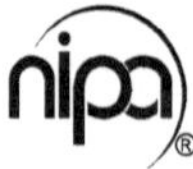

NIPA® GENX ELECTRONIC RESOURCES & SOLUTIONS P. LTD.

101,103, Vikas Surya Plaza, CU Block
L.S.C. Market, Pitam Pura, New Delhi-110 034
Ph : +91-11-43860225, Mob.: +91 9717133558, 9540816132
E-mail: newindiapublishingagency@gmail.com
Website: www.nipaersources.com

Print ISBN: 978-93-5887-987-2
ebook ISBN: 978-93-5887-303-0

Composed and Designed by NIPA®.

Preface

Agronomy and crop physiology are pivotal branches of agricultural science that focus on understanding the growth, development, and productivity of crops under varying environmental and management conditions. The integration of theoretical knowledge with practical application is essential to developing a holistic understanding of these disciplines. This lab manual, Hands-on Experiment in Agronomy and Crop Physiology is designed to bridge the gap between classroom instruction and real-world agricultural practices.

The primary objective of this manual is to provide students, researchers, and agricultural practitioners with step-by-step guidance to perform key experiments in agronomy and crop physiology. The experiments outlined in this manual have been carefully selected to cover fundamental concepts, modern methodologies, and applications essential for the study of crop science. Each experiment is structured to foster a clear understanding of the scientific principles involved, while emphasizing hands-on learning and analytical skills.

The manual is organized into chapters that encompass a wide range of topics, including soil-crop relationships, plant growth analysis, water and nutrient management, and physiological processes such as photosynthesis, transpiration, and nutrient uptake. Special attention has been given to aligning the content with current academic curricula and emerging trends in agricultural research.

To enhance the learning experience, this manual incorporates detailed protocols, illustrations, and observations sections, along with tips for accurate data collection and interpretation. Additionally, safety guidelines and precautions have been highlighted to ensure a secure and productive laboratory environment.

This manual is the result of our commitment to advancing agricultural education and research. It is intended to serve as a comprehensive resource for students pursuing degrees in agriculture, as well as for educators seeking to enrich their teaching methods.

We hope that this lab manual will inspire curiosity, foster critical thinking, and empower students to explore the dynamic field of agronomy and crop physiology. Feedback and suggestions from users are welcomed and will be invaluable in refining future editions of this manual.

Authors

Contents

Preface ..... *v*

1. Plant Nutrients 1

Terminology 1
Forms of Nutrient Elements Uptake by Plants 2
Classification of Essential Nutrients 2
Biochemical Functions of Essential Plant Nutrients 3
Based on Mobility in Plants 4

2. Physiological Functions in Crop Plants 5

Introduction 5
Nitrogen 5
Phosphurus 6
Potassium 6
Calcium 7
Magnesium 7
Sulphur 8
Iron 8
Manganese 9
Zinc 9
Copper 10
Boron 10
Molybdenum 11
Chlorine 11

3. Plant Analysis for Nutrients 13

Nitrogen 14
Phosphorus 15
Iron 15
Potassium 15
Calcium 16

4. Physiological and Agronomical Parameters 17

Partial Factor Productivity (PFP) 17
Agronomic Efficiency (AE) 17
Apparent Recovery (AR) 17
Physiological Efficiency (PE) 18

5. Importance of Soil Testing, Collection of Soil Sample, Its Processing and Handling in Laboratory 19

Why soil testing? 19
Objectives 20
Procedure for soil testing 20
Advantages of soil testing 20
Collection of representative soil sample 21
Storage 21
Precautions to be taken during collection of soil sampling 22

6. Dumas Combustion Method: A Comprehensive Analysis 25

Principle 25
Steps Involved in the Dumas Method 25
Advantages of the Dumas Method 26
Applications 26
References *26*

7. Kjeldahl Method for Determination of Nitrogen in Plant Sample 27

Principle 27
Digestion 27
Distillation 28
Titration 28
Equipment's and Apparatus 28
Reagents 28
Procedure 29
Digestion 29
Distillation 29
Titration 29
Calculation 30
Precautions 30
References *31*

8. Estimation of Phosphorus and Potassium Cations in Plant Tissue 33
Sample Digestion 33
TRI-Acid Digestion 33
Procedure 34
DI-Acid Digestion 34
Procedure 34
Phosphorus 35
Principle 35
Reagents 35
Procedure 36
Calculation 36
Potassium 37

9. Estimation of Secondary Nutrients and Micronutrient Cations in Plant Tissue 39
Sample Digestion 39
TRI-Acid Digestion 39
DI-Acid Digestion 40
Procedure 40
Calcium and Magnesium 41
Sulphur 41
Iron, Zinc, Manganese and Copper 41
Boron 41
Molybdenum 41

10. Estimation of Electrical Conductivity in Soil 43
Objective 43
Materials Required 43
Principle 43
Procedure 44
Soil Preparation 44
Preparation of Soil Extract 44
Filtration 44
Measurement of Electrical Conductivity 44
Cleaning 44
Calculation 45
Results 45
Interpretation of Results 45

Precautions 45
References 45

11. Determination of Soil pH 47

Objective 47
Materials Required 47
Principle 47
Procedure 47
Soil Preparation 47
Preparation of Soil Suspension 48
Measurement of Soil pH 48
Cleaning 48
Results 48
Interpretation of Results 48
Precautions 49
References 49

12. Estimation of Soil Organic Carbon 51

Materials Required 51
Procedure 51
Sample Preparation 51
Weighing the Soil 51
Addition of Potassium Dichromate 52
Addition of Sulfuric Acid 52
Heating (Optional) 52
Cooling the Mixture 52
Dilution 52
Addition of Indicator 52
Titration with Ferrous Ammonium Sulfate 52
Blank Titration 53
Calculations 53
Determine the Amount of Potassium Dichromate Reacted 53
Calculate the Organic Carbon Content 53
References 53

13. Determination of Chlorophyll-A, Chlorophyll-B, and Total Chlorophyll Content of Leaves Based on Fresh Weight, Dry Weight and Leaf Area 55

Procedure for Chlorophyll Extraction from Leaves 55
Sample Collection 55
Preparation of Leaf Samples 55

Homogenization ... 55
Filtration ... 56
Volume Adjustment ... 56
Spectrophotometric Measurement ... 56
Calculation of Chlorophyll Content ... 56
Repeat and Average ... 56
Precautions ... 56
References ... *57*

14. Determination of Carotenoid Content of Leaves ... 59

Introduction ... 59
Materials and Equipments ... 59
Procedure ... 59
Sample Preparation ... 59
Extraction ... 59
Preparation of Extract ... 60
Spectrophotometric Analysis ... 60
Calculation of Carotenoid Content ... 60
Repeat and Average ... 61
Points to Remember ... 61
References ... *62*

15. Determination of Leaf Relative Water Content ... 63

Materials and Equipments ... 63
Procedure ... 63
Sample Collection ... 63
Fresh Weight Measurement ... 63
Turgid Weight Measurement ... 64
Dry Weight Measurement ... 64
Calculate Relative Water Content (RWC) ... 64
Repeat Measurements ... 64
Precautions ... 64
References ... *65*

16. General Considerations of Analytical Determination ... 67

Analytical Reagents ... 67
Distilled Water ... 67
Filter Paper ... 67
Solute ... 67
Solvent ... 67
Solution ... 68

Acid ... 68
Base ... 68
pH ... 68
Concentration ... 68
Standard Solution ... 69
Saturated Solution ... 69
Unsaturated Solution ... 69
Super Saturated Solution ... 69
Molar Solution ... 69
Molal Solution ... 69
Normal Solution ... 69
Percent Solution ... 70
Reference ... *70*

17. Preparation and Standardization of Buffer Solutions for Laboratory Applications ... 71

Buffers ... 71
Mechanism of Buffer Action ... 72
Buffering Capacity ... 73
Preparation of some common Buffers ... 73
M Glycine-HCl Buffer; pH range 2.2 to 3.6 ... 73
M Hydrochloric Acid-Potassium Chloride Buffer (HCl-KCl); pH Range 1.0 to 2.2 ... 74
M Citrate Buffer; pH range 3.0 to 6.2 ... 74
M Acetate Buffer; pH range 3.6 to 5.6 ... 74
M Citrate-Phosphate Buffer; pH range 2.6 to 7.0 ... 75
Phosphate Buffer; pH range 5.8 to 8.0 ... 75
Tris-HCl Buffer, pH range 7.2 to 9.0 ... 75
Carbonate-Bicarbonate Buffer, pH range 9.2 to 10.6 ... 76

18. General Precautions for Volumetric and Gravimetric Analysis ... 77

Volumetric Analysis Precautions ... 77
Use Clean Glassware ... 77
Clean Glassware Properly ... 77
Proper Calibration ... 77
Avoid Parallax Error ... 77
Use Correct Indicators ... 77
Control Temperature ... 77
Add Reagents Slowly ... 77
Mix Solutions Thoroughly ... 77

Handle Reagents with Care 78
Gravimetric Analysis Precautions 78
Ensure Perfect Cleanliness of Apparatus 78
Dry the Sample Properly 78
Weigh Accurately 78
Avoid Contamination 78
Ensure Complete Precipitation 78
Filter and Wash Precipitates Carefully 78
Dry or Ignite Precipitates to Constant Weight 78
Avoid Loss of Material 78
Maintain a Stable Work Environment 78
References *79*

19. Study About Different Forms of Solution 81

Methods to Express Concentration of a True Solution 81
Molarity (M) 81
Molality (m) 81
Normality (N) 82
Mass Percent (% w/w) 82
Volume Percent (% v/v) 83
Mass/Volume Percent (% w/v) 83
Mole Fraction (χ) 83
Parts Per Million (ppm) and Parts Per Billion (ppb) 84
Formality (F) 84
References *85*

Plates 87

Index 93

1

Plant Nutrients

In the realm of natural elements, there exist approximately one hundred and three distinct elements. Among them, nearly ninety elements are absorbed by plants. To differentiate essential elements from those that plants can assimilate but are not vital, Arnon (1954) established the following criteria:

1. The plant must be incapable of normal growth or completing its life cycle in the absence of the element
2. The element is specific and irreplaceable by another
3. The element directly participates in plant metabolism

By applying these criteria, molybdenum and chlorine are not deemed essential, even though they serve a functional role in plant metabolism. This is because they can be substituted by vanadium and halides, respectively. Subsequently, D. J. Nicholas refined the definition of essential elements, replacing the term "functional or metabolic nutrient" to encompass any mineral element that contributes to plant metabolism, regardless of whether its action is specific.

Terminology

- **Plant nutrition:** Plant nutrition is well-defined as the supply and absorption of chemical compounds required for plant growth and metabolism.
- **Nutrients:** Nutrients are the chemical compounds or ions required by an organism for the metabolic activities and growth.
- **Beneficial elements**: Termed as potential micronutrients, these elements have not yet been definitively established as essential for growth and metabolism. However, it is believed that they may impart beneficial effects when present in extremely low concentrations. The positive impact of these nutrients may arise from their capability to influence the absorption, movement, and utilization of essential elements. Their essentiality could be specific to certain plant species or particular environmental conditions. Examples of such elements include silicon, vanadium, cobalt, and aluminum.

- **Functional elements:** Nicholas D. J. (1961) expanded the term "functional or metabolic nutrient" to encompass any mineral element participating in plant metabolism, irrespective of whether its function is specific or not.

To characterize the concentration of nutrient elements in plants, the following terms have been suggested:

1. Deficient: When an essential element is present in low concentrations that significantly restrict yield and give rise to more or less distinct deficiency symptoms.

2. Toxic: When the concentration of either an essential or other element is elevated to a level that markedly inhibits plant growth to a significant extent.

Forms of Nutrient Elements Uptake by Plants

i) Uptake as single nutrient ion ii) Uptake combined form

Element	Uptake form	Element	Uptake form
Potassium	K^+	Sodium	Na^+
Calcium	Ca^{2+}	Cobalt	Co^{2+}
Magnesium	Mg^{2+}	Sodium	Na^+
Iron	Fe^{2+}	Nitrogen	Ammonium (NH^{4+}) and Nitrate (NO^{3-})
Manganese	Mn^{2+}	Phosphorus	$H_2PO_4^-$, HPO_4^{2-}
Copper	Cu^{2+}	Sulphur	SO_4^{2-}
Zinc	Zn^{2+}	Boron	H_3BO_3, H_2BO^{3-}, HBO_3^{2-}, BO_3^{3-}
Chlorine	Cl^-	Molybdenum	MoO^{2-} (Molybdate)
Silicon	Si^{4+}	Carbon	CO_2
Cobalt	Co^{2+}	Hydrogen	H_2O

Classification of essential nutrients: Nutrients are chemical compounds essential for the growth and metabolic activities of an organism. Essential plant nutrients are categorized into macronutrients, including primary and secondary nutrients, and micronutrients.

A. Macronutrients: Macronutrients, also known as major nutrients, earn their designation due to their necessity in larger quantities by plants. These elements are present and required in comparatively higher amounts than micronutrients. The macronutrients encompass C, H, O, N, P, K, Ca, Mg and S. Notably, C, H, and O constitute 90-95% of the plant's dry matter weight, primarily sourced from carbon dioxide (CO_2) and water. The remaining six macronutrients are further classified into primary and secondary nutrients.

i) Primary nutrients: Nitrogen, phosphorus, and potassium are designated as primary nutrients due to the frequent requirement for rectifying their predominant deficiencies through the utilization of commercial fertilizers, where they serve as principal components.

ii) Secondary nutrients: Calcium, magnesium, and sulfur are classified as secondary nutrients owing to their relatively modest demand by plants, localized deficiencies, and inadvertent inclusion through carriers of primary nutrients. For instance, phosphatic fertilizers such as single super phosphate encompass both calcium and sulfur. Similarly, ammonium sulfate, a nitrogenous fertilizer, also serves as a supplementary source of sulfur.

B. Micronutrients: Micronutrients are essential elements needed by plants in relatively small quantities, yet they play crucial roles comparable to macronutrients. These elements are commonly referred to as trace elements. They can be further categorized into micronutrient cations, including iron (Fe), manganese (Mn), zinc (Zn), and copper (Cu), and micronutrient anions, consisting of boron (B), molybdenum (Mo), and chlorine (Cl), based on their available forms.

Biochemical Functions of Essential Plant Nutrients

Group 1 [C, H, O, N, S]: The principal components of organic material consist of essential elements forming atomic groups crucial for enzymatic processes and assimilation through oxidation-reduction reactions.

Group 2 [P, B, Si]: Phosphorus (P), boron (B), and silicon (Si) participate in the esterification process utilizing native alcohol groups in plants. Simultaneously, they are integral to energy transfer reactions within the biochemical pathways of the plant's cellular metabolism.

Group 3 [K, Na, Mg, Ca, Mn, Cl]: Potassium (K), sodium (Na), magnesium (Mg), calcium (Ca), manganese (Mn), and chlorine (Cl) serve diverse functions in plants, encompassing the establishment of osmotic potentials, activation of enzymes, maintenance of ion balance, regulation of membrane permeability, and modulation of electrochemical potentials within cellular processes.

Group 4 [Fe, Cu, Zn, Mo]: Iron (Fe), copper (Cu), zinc (Zn), and molybdenum (Mo) are predominantly found in a chelated form, integrated into prosthetic groups within various biological molecules.

Based on Mobility in Plant

a. **Mobile nutrients:** Mobile nutrients in plants are characterized by their ability to translocate from matured tissues, typically older leaves, to the actively growing meristem. Consequently, deficiency symptoms become apparent in the older tissue, reflecting the nutrient's movement within the plant. Eg: N, P, K, Mg

b. **Immobile nutrients:** Immobile nutrients are characterized by their incapacity to translocate from older tissues to younger ones in the event of soil deficiency. Consequently, deficiency symptoms manifest initially in the younger leaves, reflecting the nutrient's lack of mobility within the plant. Eg: Ca, B, S

2

Physiological Functions in Crop Plants

Introduction

The physiological disorder of a mineral nutrient is entirely contingent upon its function within the plant body. Inadequate or excessive supply of any essential element can result in metabolic disruptions, influencing the activities of enzymes, rates of metabolic reactions, and concentrations of metabolites. Alongside alterations in metabolic patterns, severe deficiencies of specific essential elements also give rise to distinctive effects in leaves, stems, roots, blossoms, and fruits.

A. Nitrogen

Functions: Nitrogen is essential for plants, playing crucial roles in protein synthesis, nucleic acid formation, and chlorophyll synthesis. It is a key component of enzymes, contributing to various metabolic processes. Nitrogen also supports root development, cell structure, and the synthesis of secondary metabolites. Striking a balance in nitrogen levels is vital for maintaining plant health and ensuring optimal growth and productivity. Effective nitrogen management is essential for sustainable agriculture and overall ecosystem well-being.

Deficiency symptoms: Plants displaying nitrogen levels below 1% are generally considered nitrogen deficient. The initial symptoms manifest in older leaves, characterized by a light green to pale yellow coloration due to proteolysis, a process facilitated by the high mobility of nitrogen in plants. This deficiency leads to stunted and slow growth. In grasses, lower leaves often exhibit a firing or browning pattern, starting at the leaf tip and progressing along the midrib, forming an inverted 'V' shape. Nitrogen deficiency is further associated with reduced flowering, limited tillering, slender stalks, short heads, decreased protein content, and diminished crop yields. General malnourishment and the development of anthocyanins, along with chlorosis, represent notable symptoms of nitrogen deficiency.

Toxicity symptoms: In conditions of elevated nitrogen availability, plants tend to exhibit succulence, characterized by increased water content, resulting in taller plants with heavier heads that are more susceptible to lodging. A nitrogen-rich and luxuriant crop becomes more prone to insect pest and disease attacks due to the lush and soft tissue, providing favorable conditions for such infestations.

B. Phosphurus

Functions: Phosphorus is vital for plants, serving multiple essential functions. It is crucial for energy transfer, being a key component of ATP, the primary energy carrier in cells, as well as in cellular respiration and photosynthesis. Phosphorus is also integral to nucleic acid synthesis, aiding in DNA and RNA formation, and contributes to membrane structure, enzyme activation, and root development. Additionally, phosphorus plays a role in plant stress responses. Overall, maintaining adequate phosphorus levels is essential for optimal plant growth, development, and productivity.

Deficiency symptoms: Plants with phosphorus levels below 0.1% are generally classified as phosphorus-deficient. Given its relatively rapid mobility within plants, phosphorus is translocated from older tissues to meristematic tissues. Consequently, the initial symptoms of phosphorus deficiency manifest on the older leaves of young plants. Phosphorus-deficient plants exhibit dark green leaves, stunted growth, thin and erect structures with sparse and restricted foliage, and severe limitations in root development. Lateral bud production is suppressed, foliage may appear bluish green, and prolonged deficiency can lead to bronzing or reddish-purple tips or margins on older leaves due to the accumulation of sugars that stimulate anthocyanin synthesis. Additionally, leaf tips may brown and die in some cases.

Toxicity symptoms: An excessive presence of phosphorus (P) can induce a deficiency of trace elements such as iron (Fe) and zinc (Zn) in plants. This is attributed to the complex interactions and interferences that high levels of phosphorus can have on the availability and uptake of these essential trace elements, leading to imbalances and potential deficiencies in the plant.

C. Potassium

Functions: Potassium is essential for various physiological functions in plants. It plays a crucial role in regulating water uptake and retention, enhancing drought tolerance and osmotic regulation. Potassium is also involved in enzyme activation, facilitating numerous biochemical reactions crucial for plant metabolism and growth. Additionally, potassium regulates stomatal opening and closing, influencing gas exchange and water loss. It contributes to photosynthesis by aiding in the transport of sugars and enhancing plant energy production. Furthermore, potassium supports the synthesis of proteins and nucleic acids, contributing to overall plant development and stress resistance.

Deficiency symptoms: Potassium (K) deficiency in plants may initially manifest as hidden hunger, where visible symptoms are not immediately apparent. The deficiency is characterized by a reduction in growth rate, chlorosis (yellowing of leaves), and, in later stages, necrosis (cell death). The first signs of deficiency typically appear on the older leaves. As the deficiency progresses, gradual chlorosis along the leaf margins occurs, followed by scorching and browning of the tips of older leaves, giving them a burnt appearance. The plant experiences slow and stunted growth, and there is an increased risk of crop lodging.

Toxicity symptoms: Potassium (K) toxicity can lead to cation imbalance, resulting in reduced uptake and subsequent deficiencies of magnesium (Mg), and in certain instances, calcium (Ca). The excess of potassium can disrupt the proper uptake and utilization of these essential cations, leading to imbalances in plant nutrition.

D. Calcium

Calcium plays a crucial role as an integral component of plant cell walls, actively participating in the regulation of cell wall construction. Typically, soils are naturally abundant in calcium. Deficiency symptoms are not evident as long as the soil pH is maintained within the neutral range. However, calcium deficiency is characterized by a reduction in meristematic tissue. Insufficient calcium can lead to the distortion of young leaves, which exhibit an abnormal dark green coloration. Leaf tips often become dry or brittle, eventually withering and dying. Additionally, stems may become weak, and poor germination can be observed in plants deficient in calcium.

E. Magnesium

Functions: Magnesium (Mg) stands as a vital nutrient crucial for a diverse range of fundamental physiological and biochemical processes in plants. Its roles encompass the synthesis of chlorophyll, the production, transportation, and utilization of photo assimilates, as well as the activation of enzymes and synthesis of proteins.

Deficiency symptoms: Magnesium (Mg) is a mobile element, easily translocating from older to younger plant parts, resulting in the manifestation of deficiency symptoms initially in the older leaves. Plants experiencing magnesium deficiency typically exhibit levels below 0.1% Mg. This deficiency is commonly observed in plants cultivated in coarse-textured acidic soils.

F. Sulphur

Functions: Sulphur is vital for various growth functions in plants, encompassing nitrogen metabolism, enzyme activity, and the synthesis of proteins and oils. Typically, plants deficient in sulphur exhibit stunted and/or slender stems, along with yellowing of the young (top) leaves. In contrast to nitrogen deficiency, where yellowing primarily affects the older, lower leaves first.

Deficiency symptoms: The sulphur content in plant tissues typically falls within the range of 0.1 to 0.4%. In India, sulphur deficiency is prevalent, positioning sulfur as the fourth most deficient major nutrient, following nitrogen (N), phosphorus (P), and potassium (K). Plants experiencing sulfur deficiency tend to accumulate non-protein nitrogen, primarily in the form of nitrate and amide. The nitrogen-to-sulfur (N:S) ratio in plants typically spans from 9 to 12:1. Due to its immobility within the plant, sulphur deficiency manifests first in young leaves.

G. Iron

Functions: Iron is a vital micronutrient for plants, serving essential functions in various metabolic processes. One of its primary roles is in chlorophyll synthesis, the green pigment critical for photosynthesis. Iron is also involved in electron transport chains, playing a crucial role in energy transfer within plant cells. Additionally, iron is a cofactor for enzymes involved in the reduction of nitrates and sulfates, influencing nitrogen and sulfur metabolism. Iron contributes to the activation of enzymes responsible for DNA and RNA synthesis, essential for genetic processes in plants. Maintaining proper iron levels is crucial for overall plant health, as it impacts growth, development, and the plant's ability to cope with environmental stressors.

Deficiency symptoms: The critical threshold for iron in plants is 30 ppm, with a sufficiency range of 50 to 250 ppm. Iron deficiency leads to reduced chlorophyll production, resulting in interveinal chlorosis characterized by yellowing between leaf veins, particularly noticeable in young leaves. As deficiency progresses, affected leaves may exhibit tip and margin burn, spreading inward, eventually leading to widespread leaf necrosis and tissue death. Leaves may turn white as chlorophyll diminishes, causing them to fall off along with twigs. Lime-induced chlorosis is another symptom resulting from iron deficiency.

Toxicity symptoms: Toxic conditions typically arise in acidic soils (pH<5.0) or when excessive soluble iron salts are used as foliar sprays or soil amendments. Soil with high iron concentrations usually does not cause injury in neutral or high pH environments, except in cases of saturation, poor drainage, compaction, or inadequate aeration. Iron toxicity is also more likely when zinc levels are low.

H. Manganese

Functions: Manganese is essential for plants, acting as a cofactor for enzymes in photosynthesis, aiding chlorophyll synthesis and electron transfer. It also scavenges reactive oxygen species, reducing oxidative stress and protecting plant cells. Manganese facilitates nitrogen and carbohydrate metabolism, contributing to growth and development. Crucially, it supports amino acid and protein synthesis, vital for plant structure and function. Overall, manganese is crucial for maintaining plant health, photosynthesis, and stress resilience.

Deficiency symptoms: Manganese deficiency in plants, indicated by manganese levels below 25 ppm, leads to chlorosis in young leaves. Unlike iron deficiency, the chlorosis appears diffuse without clear vein distinctions. Dicotyledonous plants show chlorotic and necrotic spots between veins, while monocotyledonous plants, like cereals, exhibit greenish-grey spots, flecks, and stripes on basal leaves (Grey speck). As deficiency progresses, chlorotic areas turn red, reddish-brown, or brown.

Toxicity symptoms: Manganese toxicity typically presents with blackish-brown or red spots on older leaves, along with an irregular distribution of chlorophyll, resulting in chlorosis and necrotic lesions.

I. Zinc

Functions: Zinc is essential for plants, acting as a cofactor for enzymes involved in DNA replication, protein synthesis, and chlorophyll formation. It supports hormone regulation, root development, and stress response mechanisms. Overall, zinc is crucial for maintaining healthy growth, development, and stress resilience in plants.

Deficiency symptoms: Zinc exhibits intermediate mobility within plants, with symptoms typically appearing first in middle leaves. Chlorotic areas may vary in color, ranging from pale green to yellow or white. Severe zinc deficiency can result in leaves turning gray-white and premature leaf fall or death. Affected plants often display significant stunting, with limited flowering and seed set.

Toxicity symptoms: Toxicity from zinc is infrequent but can arise in highly saline soils. Symptoms include dark green leaves, chlorosis, interveinal chlorosis, and a decrease in both root growth and leaf expansion. Additionally, excess zinc may trigger iron deficiency in plants.

J. Copper

Functions: In plants, copper is essential for a variety of vital functions, such as electron transport, photosynthesis, and respiration, which facilitate energy production and metabolism. It is also an essential component of the formation and strengthening of plant cell walls, which contributes to the rigidity and structure of the plant. Copper is also involved in the synthesis of lignin, a key component of cell walls, and in the regulation of hormone levels, affecting plant development and growth.

Deficiency symptoms: Plants with copper levels below 5 ppm are deemed copper deficient, displaying distinct symptoms such as chlorosis in younger shoot tissue, leaf distortion, tip whitening, and dieback. Copper deficiency may also result in "reclamation disease," characterized by poor growth. Notably, copper deficiency can lead to male flower sterility, delayed flowering, and premature aging. In dicots, the cessation of shoot apex growth triggers the proliferation of auxiliary buds, while in cereals, necrosis of the apical meristem prompts shoot elongation, often accompanied by bleaching and wilting of young leaves.

Toxicity symptoms: Copper toxicity in plants can lead to stunted growth, root damage, chlorosis, leaf distortion, and reduced reproductive capacity. It may also disrupt nutrient uptake, impacting overall plant health and productivity.

K. Boron

Functions: Boron is essential for numerous vital functions in plants, including cell wall formation, nutrient uptake, carbohydrate metabolism, hormone synthesis, and flower development. It plays a crucial role in maintaining structural integrity, facilitating nutrient transport, and regulating growth processes. Additionally, boron contributes to water balance regulation and reproductive success. Overall, boron is indispensable for optimal plant growth and development.

Deficiency symptoms: Plants with boron concentrations ranging from 5 to 30 ppm are considered boron deficient. However, the critical deficiency range varies, from 5 to 10 ppm in gramineous plants to 20 to 70 ppm in dicotyledons. Boron deficiency is characterized by chlorotic young leaves and the death of the terminal bud. Brittle and distorted leaves and stems, along with thickened and curled leaf tips due to disrupted cell wall growth, are common symptoms. Stunted growth, resulting from shortened internodes, gives affected plants a bushy or rosette-like appearance.

Toxicity symptoms: Boron toxicity in plants typically initiates with chlorosis, leading to necrosis. Symptoms first emerge at the leaf tips and margins, spreading towards the midrib as toxicity advances. With continued exposure, older leaves may exhibit scorching and premature shedding.

L. Molybdenum

Functions: Molybdenum plays crucial roles in various metabolic processes within plants. As a cofactor for enzymes such as nitrogenase and nitrate reductase, molybdenum facilitates nitrogen fixation and nitrate assimilation, essential processes for plant growth and development. It is also involved in the conversion of inorganic phosphorus into organic forms, aiding in phosphorus metabolism. Additionally, molybdenum participates in the synthesis of certain amino acids, particularly those involved in nitrogen metabolism, and helps regulate plant responses to stress, including drought and salinity.

Deficiency symptoms: The initial sign of molybdenum deficiency in many plants is the appearance of reticulate venation, characterized by prominent chlorotic mottling between the veins. Molybdenum deficiency can also lead to the accumulation of nitrates in plants. In legumes, symptoms resemble those of nitrogen deficiency, while grasses generally have lower molybdenum requirements.

Toxicity symptoms: Toxicity from molybdenum in plants typically presents with symptoms such as leaf chlorosis and necrosis. Initially, chlorosis may appear between leaf veins, gradually spreading to the entire leaf surface. As toxicity progresses, necrotic lesions may develop, leading to tissue death. Additionally, excess molybdenum can disrupt nutrient uptake and metabolism, resulting in overall plant stunting and reduced growth.

M. Chlorine

Functions: Chlorine plays essential roles in plant physiology, primarily in maintaining osmotic balance, stomatal regulation, and photosynthesis. It helps regulate osmotic pressure within plant cells, ensuring proper water uptake and nutrient transport. Furthermore, chlorine contributes to the photosynthetic process by participating in the water-splitting reaction during the light-dependent phase.

Deficiency symptoms: Chlorine deficiency in plants typically manifests as a wilted appearance in foliage and root systems, with lateral roots exhibiting branching. Prominent symptoms in crops include chlorosis, mottling, bronzing, and tissue necrosis in the leaves.

Toxicity symptoms: While chlorine is required in trace amounts for plant growth, excessive levels can lead to toxicity, resulting in leaf burn, wilting, and reduced photosynthetic efficiency. Overall, chlorine is vital for maintaining proper cellular function and optimizing plant growth and development. Other symptoms include decrease in leaf number and size, as well as burning, scorching, or firing of leaf tips and margins. Bronzing, premature yellowing, and shedding of leaves are also common indicators. In some cases, growth reduction may occur without any visible leaf symptoms.

3

Plant Analysis for Nutrients

The growth and productivity of crops depend on various factors, with the nutrient content of plant parts like leaves and stems playing a crucial role. These parts are often used as indicators to assess the nutrient status of plants. Each crop requires essential elements at specific concentrations during different growth stages, known as 'critical levels'. When the nutrient content falls below these critical levels, plants may display symptoms of deficiency.

Nutrient requirements and availability can be evaluated through: i) plant diagnosis, ii) soil analysis, and iii) plant analysis using qualitative or quantitative methods. By conducting these tests, necessary nutrients can be identified and applied to crops to sustain growth and correct deficiencies. While rapid tissue tests offer quick solutions for nutritional problems, quantitative estimation of both plant and soil nutrient concentrations is more economical and provides a long-term strategy for managing nutritional issues. Implementing quantitative estimation allows for informed application of fertilizers, whether as basal or foliar, thus addressing deficiencies effectively and ensuring sustainable crop growth.

Plant analysis consists of two methods:

1. Tissue testing
2. Whole plant analysis

Rapid tissue test: This method involves a rapid and semi-quantitative assessment of nutrient levels in plants. Fresh plant tissue or sap extracted from ruptured cells is utilized for testing unassimilated N, P, K, and other essential nutrients. By adding specific reagents, color development occurs in the cell sap. The intensity of the resulting color is then categorized as low, medium, or high, indicating nutrient deficiencies, adequacy, or abundance in the plants, respectively. This approach primarily serves to predict nutrient deficiencies and can help anticipate certain production challenges.

Whole plant analysis: This quantitative method involves analyzing either whole plants or specific plant parts. Dried plant material undergoes digestion with acid mixtures and is then subjected to various quantitative testing methods to determine nutrient concentrations. This analysis provides information on both assimilated and unassimilated nutrients, including nitrogen, phosphorus, potassium, calcium, magnesium, sulfur, iron, manganese, copper, boron, molybdenum, cobalt, chlorine, silicon, zinc, aluminum, and others. For precise results, recently matured plant material is preferred.

Table 1: The nutrient status of various elements on dry weight basis as listed below:

N - 1-3.0%	Fe - 10-50 ppm	Cl - 0.2-2.0 ppm
P - 0.05-1.0%	Cu - 1 ppm	S - 0.2-0.5 ppm
K - 0.8-1.0%	Mo - 0.05-0.35 ppm	Cu - 5-20 ppm
Ca - 0.3-0.5%	Zn - 15-20 ppm	Mo - 1.0-2.0 ppm
Mg - 0.2-0.3%	B - 6-15 ppm	

Table 2: The nutrient and reagents used for test are listed below:

Nutrient	Reagent
Nitrogen	1% diphenylamine in conc. Sulphuric acid
Phosphorus	**i. Ammonium molybdate solution-** 8 g of Ammonium molybdate is dissolved in 100 ml of distilled water. To this add 126 ml of conc. Hydrochloric acid (HCl) and volume is made upto 300 ml with distilled water. This stock solution is kept in an amber colored bottle; at the time of use, it is taken and diluted in the ratio of 1:4 using distilled water **ii. Stannous chloride powder**
Iron	Conc. H_2SO_4, conc. HNO_3, Ammonium thiocyanate and Amyl alcohol
Potassium	**i.** Sodium cobalt nitrate reagent- Take 5 gm cobalt nitrate and mix with 30 gm of sodium nitrate in 80ml of distilled water. To this, 5ml of glacial acetic acid is added. The volume is made up to 100 ml distilled water. Dilute reagent prepared (5 ml) with 15 mg sodium nitrate to 100 ml using distilled water **ii. Ethyl alcohol** (95%)
Calcium	**Morgan's Reagent:** 30 ml of glacial acetic acid and 100 grams of sodium acetate are dissolved in a little of distilled water

1. Nitrogen

Procedure- A small amount of leaf or petiole is placed in a petri dish, and a drop of 1% diphenylamine solution is added. The appearance of a blue color indicates the presence of nitrate-nitrogen. The intensity of the color reflects the amount of nitrogen present in the leaf sample.

Dark blue: sufficient

Light blue: slightly deficient

No colour: highly deficient

2. Phosphorus

Procedure- A teaspoon of freshly chopped leaf bits is placed in a test tube, and 10 ml of ammonium molybdate reagent is added. After allowing it to stand for a few minutes, the mixture is shaken, and a pinch of stannous chloride is introduced. The resulting color change is then observed.

Dark blue: sufficient

Bluish green: slightly deficient

No colour: highly deficient

3. Iron

Procedure- 0.5 grams of finely cut leaf material is placed in a glass vial, followed by the addition of 1 ml of concentrated HCl. After 15 minutes, 10 ml of distilled water and 2-3 drops of concentrated HNO_3 are added. Two minutes later, 10 ml of this solution is transferred to a specimen tube, and 5 ml of 20% ammonium thiocyanate is added and stirred. Subsequently, 2 ml of amyl alcohol is added, the mixture is shaken well, and allowed to stand for a few minutes. The intensity of the red color in the amyl alcohol layer indicates the quantity of iron present.

Brick red: sufficient Fe

Faint color: deficient Fe

4. Potassium

Procedure- Finely chopped leaf bits are placed in a test tube, and 10 ml of diluted reagent is added. The mixture is shaken vigorously for a few minutes and left to stand for 5 minutes. Subsequently, 5 ml of ethyl alcohol reagent is added, and the solution is allowed to stand for 3 minutes. Finally, the solution is observed for the formation of turbidity.

Turbidity: sufficient K

Less turbidity: slightly deficient K

5. Calcium

Procedure- In a glass vial, 0.5 g of finely cut plant material is taken from both a healthy plant and a deficient plant, each in separate vials. To each vial, 5 ml of Morgan's reagent is added. After allowing it to stand for 15 minutes, 2 ml of glycerin and 5 ml of 10% ammonium oxalate are added to each solution. The mixture is then shaken for 2 minutes. The turbidity observed after 15 minutes indicates the amount of calcium present in the normal plant tissue.

4

Physiological and Agronomical Parameters

The seed yield, along with the rate of application and uptake of nutrients, is used to determine the following parameters for nitrogen or other nutrients:

Partial Factor Productivity (PFP) (kg seed/kg N applied): Partial Factor Productivity (PFP) is a measure used in agriculture to assess the efficiency of nutrient use, particularly nitrogen or other essential nutrients, in crop production. It is calculated as the ratio of the seed yield to the rate of nutrient application. The formula for PFP is:

$$\text{PFP} = \frac{\text{Seed Yield}}{\text{Rate of Nutrient Application}}$$

*A higher PFP value indicates greater efficiency, meaning that more crop yield is produced per unit of nutrient applied. This is desirable as it implies that the nutrient is being used more effectively by the crop.

Agronomic Efficiency (AE) (kg seed/kg N applied): Agronomic Efficiency is a measure used to evaluate the effectiveness of nutrient application in increasing crop yield. It specifically assesses the yield gain per unit of nutrient applied. The formula for AE is:

$$\text{AE} = \frac{\text{Increase in Yield due to Nutrient Application}}{\text{Rate of Nutrient Application}}$$

*A higher AE value indicates that the nutrient application is highly effective in increasing crop yield. This means that each unit of nutrient applied results in a substantial yield gain.

Apparent Recovery (AR) (kg N uptake/kg N applied): Apparent Recovery also known as Recovery Efficiency (RE), is a measure used in agriculture to determine the proportion of applied nutrients that are taken up by the crop. It reflects how effectively a crop utilizes the applied nutrients. The formula for

AR is:

$$AR = \frac{\text{Increase in Nutrient Uptake}}{\text{Rate of Nutrient Application}} \times 100$$

*A higher AR value indicates that a larger proportion of the applied nutrient is being absorbed by the crop. This suggests efficient nutrient use and good nutrient uptake conditions.

Physiological Efficiency (PE) (kg seed/kg of N removed): Physiological Efficiency is a measure used in agriculture to evaluate the effectiveness of the absorbed nutrients in enhancing crop yield. It focuses on the yield increase per unit of nutrient taken up by the plant. The formula for PE is:

$$PE = \frac{\text{Increase in Yield due to Nutrient Application}}{\text{Increase in Nutrient Uptake}}$$

*A higher PE value indicates that the nutrient taken up by the crop is being used very effectively to increase yield. This means that for each unit of nutrient absorbed, there is a significant yield gain.

5

Importance of Soil Testing, Collection of Soil Sample, Its Processing and Handling in Laboratory

Assessment of a soil's fertility status involves an estimation of its available nutrient status i.e., the portion or amount of nutrient directly available in soil for subsequent uptake by crop plant. This exercise commonly referred to as soil testing and is used to arrive at optimum fertilizer application ratio. The need for estimation of available nutrient arises because only a small fraction of what the soil contains is the total nutrient content of the soil. Soil test is calibrated by correlating them with crop response and the result from the basis for making fertilizer recommendations.

Estimation of nutrient contents and forms in materials that are involved in nutrient supply and dynamics is a conical step towards planning scientific nutrient management. In this content, both soil and plant testing information come out of the interpretation of analysis assumes a greater value when their concentrations and amounts can relate to soil fertility, nutrient availability, plant growth, yield and quality of the crop produce.

Why soil testing?

- Soil fertility status assessment involves an estimation of its available nutrient status.
- It gives the amount of nutrient directly available in soil for subsequent uptake by crop plant.
- Guides to arrive at optimum fertilizer application.
- It is a method of evaluating nutrient status (physico-chemical properties) of the soil i.e., the assessment of the fertility of the soil to determine nutrient deficiencies.
- It is also concerned with environmental quality for the community hazards.

Objectives

(i) To evaluate soil fertility and its productivity by the estimation of level of nutrients (Low, Medium, High)

(ii) Grouping of soil for their classification

(iii) To determine the specific soil problem such as an acidity (H^+ or Al^{3+}), alkalinity (Na^+, Ca^{2+}, Mg^{2+}, K^+) and sodicity (sodium ions) if exist. Subsequently giving recommendations for their correction (Lime/ Gypsum requirement etc.)

(iv) To predict the probability of getting maximum response of crops to fertilizers

Procedure for soil testing

The procedure for testing the soil to meet these objectives is divided into the following phases:

(i) Collection of soil samples and its preparation

(ii) Extraction and determination of nutrients and physico-chemical properties of the soil

(iii) Interpretation of analytical results

(iv) Recommendation and follow up of results and evaluation of recommendations

Soil testing is a chemical method for estimation of nutrient supplying power of a soil/ soil fertility evaluation. Soil fertility may be defined as the capacity of soil to furnish available plant nutrients to the plants in proper amount and appropriate balance, under ideal condition of plant growth.

Advantages of soil testing

- More rapid method as compare to biological or deficiency symptoms/ plant analysis.
- One may determine the need of the soil before the planting of crop.
- To determine the suitability of the soil for laying gardens.
- Soil survey.

Apparatus and materials: Khurpi, Spade, Augers, Plastic bowl, Scale, Rack, Wooden roller, Mortar and pestle, Sieve, Polythene/paper/cloth bags, Labels, Card board cartons, Aluminium boxes

Collection of representative soil sample

- Based on difference in soil type, colour, crop growth or slope, divide the area in different homogenous units.
- In the uniform field, demarked the sampling points in a zig zag fashion or randomly in such a way that the whole field should be covered. This way, soils from 8-10 places depending on the area should be collected and mixed uniformly.
- The waste material like grasses, leaves, etc. should be removed from the surface.
- If the soils are hard, make a 'V' shape cut upto 15 cm depth. Remove the soil of the pit. Now scrap or remove 1 cm soil from the surface upto 15 cm depth from both the side with the help of khurpi. This scraped soil is collected in a plastic bowl. This sample is known as 'primary' sample. Such primary samples should be approximately the same weight.
- After collecting at least 8-10 primary samples, mix all the samples in plastic bowl thoroughly and draw about ½ kg composite sample by quartering method. Label the sample in the bowl and divide the sample in approximately 4 equal parts. Discard the 2 opposite portions of the samples and remaining 2 portions are again thoroughly mixed and again divided in to 4 equal parts and 2 opposite parts again discarded. This procedure is continued until ½ kg sample remain in the bowl. This is known as composite sample which is true representative of the area.
- The most suitable containers for soil samples are polythene bags 6 x 9" made of film about 0.13 mm thick, which may be sealed by twisting or tying the neck or by mean of rubber bands or adhesive tape.
- If the soil is to be kept in moist condition for moisture determination, bacterial count and nitrate estimation etc. air tight containers are preferred.

Storage

- The registered and labelled samples in laboratory are finally placed in a cardboard carton.
- Label the carton properly with the details of soil sample and store in a separate room.

- The room should be away from direct sunlight/wind or dampness.
- The room exposed to heat or cold or dampness in not advisable.

Precautions to be taken during collection of soil sampling

1. Remove all debris from surface before collection of soil sample.
2. Avoid taking sample from upland and low land areas in the same field.
3. Take separate sample from the areas of different appearances.
4. In row crop take sample in between rows.
5. Keep the sample in a clean bag.
6. A sample should not be taken from large area (more than 1-2 ha).
7. Sample for micronutrient analysis must be collected by steel or rust free khurpi/auger and kept in clean polythene bag.
8. Avoid sampling from low – lying spots, manure dumping sites, near trees and from fertilizer placed zones.
9. Use clean bags for sample collection. Do not use bags which had earlier contained fertilizer, manure or plant protection chemicals etc.
10. A single field can be heterogeneous or variable thus soil sampling should be done considering this.
11. Based on the soil colour, slope, depth, crop type, salinity, sodicity, etc. separate sample should be collected.
12. To get accurate soil testing analysis, avoid sampling from the following places: farmyard manure applied places, chemical fertilizer applied places, near bund areas, waterlogged areas, below tree areas, near cattle shed areas, etc.
13. Simple equipments- spade, weeding hoe, etc. should be used for soil sampling.
14. Avoid use do the metal instruments, if testing of the soil for micronutrients has to be done. Use the wood instrument in these cases.
15. In general, one soil sample for 1.5 to 2.0 acre or 0.5 ha land should be collected.
16. The soil sample should be collected after the harvesting of the crop or before sowing or planting or before onset of monsoon or before application of the fertilizers.

17. In standing crop, the soil sample should be collected in between two rows of the crops.

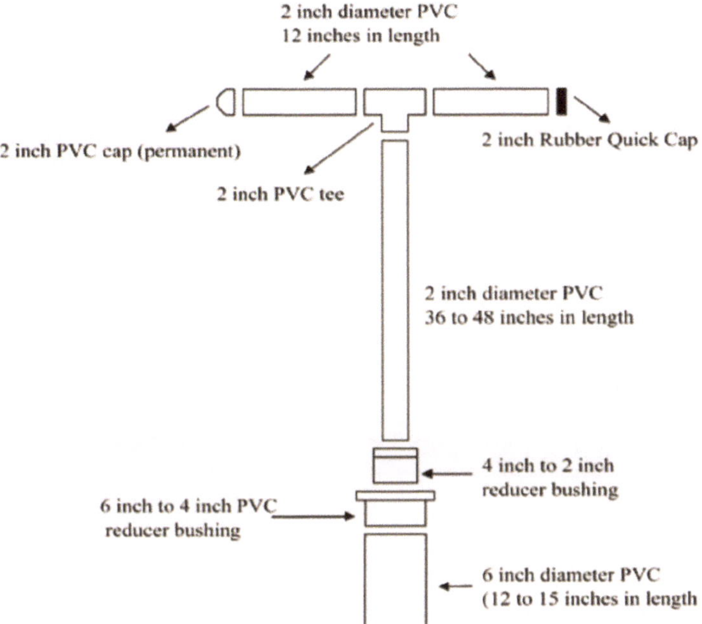

Fig. 1. Core Sampler

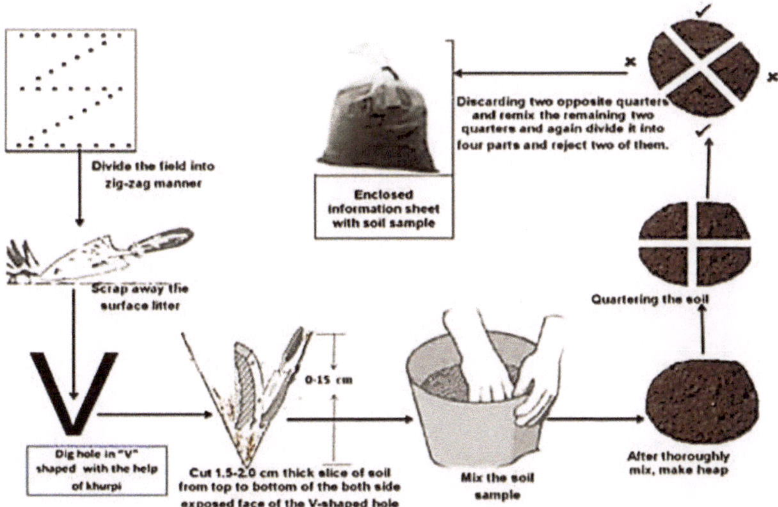

Fig. 2: Schematics on the scientific soil sampling procedure

6

Dumas Combustion Method A Comprehensive Analysis

The Dumas combustion method, named after the renowned French chemist Jean-Baptiste Dumas, is a widely recognized analytical technique employed in the determination of the elemental composition of organic compounds. This method involves the complete combustion of a sample in an oxygen-rich environment, followed by the separation and subsequent analysis of the resulting combustion products.

Principle

The Dumas combustion method involves the complete combustion of a sample in the presence of excess oxygen. The nitrogen present in the organic compound is converted into nitrogen gas (N_2), which is then measured quantitatively. The process can be summarized as follows:

i. **Combustion**: The sample is combusted at high temperatures (typically around 900-1000°C) in the presence of oxygen. This results in the conversion of all organic material into carbon dioxide (CO_2), water (H_2O), and nitrogen gas (N_2).

ii. **Removal of Interfering Gases**: The combustion products are passed through various reagents to remove interfering gases such as CO_2 and H_2O.

iii. **Detection of Nitrogen**: The nitrogen gas is then measured, often using a thermal conductivity detector (TCD) or another suitable detection method.

Steps Involved in the Dumas Method

i. **Sample Preparation**: The sample, typically a few milligrams, is accurately weighed and placed in a combustion tube.

ii. **Combustion**: The sample is combusted in an oxygen-rich environment. This can be done using an automatic analyzer, where the sample is introduced into a high-temperature furnace.

iii. **Gas Purification**: The gases produced are passed through a series of traps or reagents to remove CO_2 and H_2O, leaving only N_2.

iv. **Detection and Quantification**: The purified nitrogen gas is then measured using a suitable detector. The amount of nitrogen is directly proportional to the nitrogen content of the sample.

Advantages of the Dumas Method

- **Speed:** The Dumas method is relatively quick, often taking only a few minutes per sample.
- **Accuracy and Precision:** It provides accurate and precise measurements of nitrogen content.
- **No Use of Hazardous Chemicals:** Unlike the Kjeldahl method, the Dumas method does not require the use of hazardous chemicals like sulfuric acid and mercury.
- **Automation:** The process can be fully automated, reducing the potential for human error and increasing throughput.

Applications

- **Agricultural Sciences**: Used for determining the protein content in grains, soil, and plant tissues.
- **Food Industry**: Employed to measure the protein content in food products.
- **Biochemical Research**: Used to analyze the nitrogen content in biological samples.
- **Environmental Monitoring**: Helps in the analysis of nitrogen in environmental samples such as soil and water.

References

AOAC International (2019). *Official Methods of Analysis of AOAC International*, 21st Edition.

Gutknecht, J., & Frank, E. H. (2017). "Nitrogen determination by Dumas combustion method: challenges and opportunities." *Journal of Analytical Science and Technology*, 8(1), 11.

Nelson, D. W., & Sommers, L. E. (1980). "Total Nitrogen Analysis of Soil and Plant Tissues." *Journal of the Association of Official Analytical Chemists*, 63, 770-778.

7

Kjeldahl Method for Determination of Nitrogen in Plant Sample

Nitrogen, a key component of organic materials like proteins, is analyzed using the Kjeldahl method, which is the global standard for determining protein content in various substances, including human and animal foods, fertilizers, wastewater, and fossil fuels. The Kjeldahl method involves three main steps:

A. Digestion

B. Distillation

C. Titration

Nitrogen, making up 1-4% of a plant's dry weight, is vital for synthesizing chlorophyll, proteins, and other key compounds. Plants with high nitrogen levels turn dark green due to increased chlorophyll. Understanding nitrogen content in plant tissues is crucial for diagnosing deficiencies or toxicity and for effective nutrient management to improve crop production.

Determining the nitrogen content in plants is crucial for understanding plant nutrition, assessing the efficiency of fertilizer use, and making informed decisions in agricultural practices. Various methods can be used to determine nitrogen in plant tissues, with the most common ones being the Kjeldahl method, the Dumas method, and near-infrared reflectance spectroscopy (NIRS).

Principle

Organic nitrogen in plant tissues is converted to ammonium sulfate by digestion with concentrated sulfuric acid. The ammonium is then distilled as ammonia after neutralizing the solution with a strong base. The amount of ammonia is quantified by titration, which reflects the total nitrogen content in the sample.

Digestion

In the Kjeldahl method, plant samples are digested by boiling with concentrated sulfuric acid (H_2SO_4), as nitric acid (HNO_3) is unsuitable for this process. Catalysts like mercury (Hg), copper (Cu), or selenium (Se) speed up the digestion, and salts such as potassium sulfate (K_2SO_4) or sodium sulfate (Na_2SO_4) increase the temperature. During digestion, organic materials decompose, converting carbon to CO_2, oxygen to H_2O, and nitrogen to ammonia (NH_3), which then reacts with H_2SO_4 to form ammonium sulfate ($(NH_4)_2SO_4$). This process prevents the volatilization of ammonia.

Distillation

During the digestion stage, the ammonium sulphate produced releases NH_3 under strong alkaline condition created by NaOH during distillation stage. The liberated NH_3 reacts with H_2O and is converted to ammonium hydroxide and finally absorbed in boric acid by forming ammonium tetra borate.

Titration

The amount of ammonia collected is determined by titration with a standard base (such as sodium hydroxide, NaOH). The volume of titrant used allows for the calculation of nitrogen content in the sample. The volume of H_2SO_4 required will be equivalent to the ammonium tetra borate formed and is a measure of N content of the plant sample.

Equipment's and Apparatus

Kjeldahl digestion assembly, ammonia distillation assembly, Kjeldahl flasks, conical flasks or beaker, pipette, burette, etc.

Reagents

1. Concentrated H_2SO_4
2. 0.1 N H_2SO_4: Dilute 2.8 ml of conc. H_2SO_4 to 1000 ml with distilled water and standardize it against standard Na_2CO_3 solution.
3. Digestion mixture: Mix 25.0 g of K_2SO_4, 5 g of $CuSO_4$. $5H_2O$ and 0.5 g of metallic selenium by grinding in a mortar.
4. 40% NaOH solution: Dissolve 400 g of NaOH in about 800 ml distilled water and make up the volume to 1000 ml.
5. 0.1 N Sodium Carbonate: Dissolve 0.530 g of anhydrous Na_2CO_3in about 20 ml redistilled water and dilute the contents to 100 ml mark in volumetric flask.
6. 2% Boric acid indicator solution: Dissolve 20 g of boric acid in about 900 ml of hot water. Cool and add 20 ml of mixed indicator solution

(prepared by dissolving 0.1 g of bromocresol green and 0.07 g of methyl red in 100 ml of ethanol). Add 0.1 M NaOH solution dropwise until the color is reddish purple and dilute to 1 L with distilled water.

Procedure

Digestion

1. Weigh 0.5 g to 1 g of processed sample of homogenized plant tissue in Kjeldahl.
2. Add 25 ml of conc. H_2SO_4 and let it stand for 30 minutes. Similarly, run a blank in another 800 ml Kjeldahl flask.
3. After half an hour of adding conc. H_2SO_4, add 5 g of the digestion mixture.
4. Place the flask in digestion unit and digest the content at low heat to prevent frothing.
5. After about 15-20 minutes gradually raise the temperature until the content become clear and colored pale green or blue.

Distillation

1. Cool the contents and add about 50 ml of distilled water and swirl the flask for about 2 minutes and take the supernatant liquid into a distillation flask.
2. Add 50 ml of 0.32% $KMNO_4$ and 50 ml of 40% NaOH along with one spoon of paraffin wax (1-2 g).
3. In the receiving end of the distillation unit, keep a 250 ml conical flask containing 20 ml 2% boric acid indicator solution to collect the released ammonia.
4. Start distillation by using automatic distillation unit for 9-12 minutes until about 100 ml of distillate is collected.
5. Pinkish colour turns to light green by the absorption of ammonia.
6. Run a blank without sample in the same manner.

Titration

The boric acid solution used in distillation is titrated with 0.1 N H_2SO_4. Change of green colour back to original pink colour indicates the end point of titration.

Calculation

$$\text{Nitrogen (\%)} = \left(\frac{V_{acid} \times N_{acid} \times 14}{W_{sample}}\right) \times 100$$

Where, V_{acid} = Volume of acid used in the titration (in ml)

N_{acid} = Normality of the acid used for titration

14 = Atomic weight of nitrogen

W_{sample} = Weight of the sample (in grams)

Note

- N content of plant samples may vary from < 1.0% to even more than 4.0% depending upon the plant species, and the plant parts analysed.
- When no more NH_3 will evolve, test with a wet red litmus paper not turning blue.
- It is desirable to use redistilled water, if distilled water is found to be distinctly alkaline.

By applying this formula, you can determine the percentage of nitrogen present in the sample. To calculate the protein content, this nitrogen value is often multiplied by a conversion factor, typically 6.25, based on the assumption that proteins contain about 16% nitrogen.

$\text{Protein (\%)} = \text{Nitrogen(\%)} \times 6.25$

Precautions

- Wear safety goggles, gloves, and a lab coat when handling concentrated sulfuric acid and catalysts.
- Perform digestion and handling of chemicals in a well-ventilated fume hood.
- Carefully add sodium hydroxide to avoid splattering and foaming.
- Ensure airtightness to prevent loss of ammonia gas.
- Digest until a clear solution is obtained to ensure full nitrogen release.

References

AOAC International (2019). *Official Methods of Analysis of AOAC International*, 21st Edition.

Kjeldahl, J. (1883). "A New Method for the Determination of Nitrogen in Organic Bodies." *Zeitschrift für Analytische Chemie*, 22, 366–383.

Miller, R. O., & Kissel, D. E. (2010). "Comparison of Soil Nitrogen Analysis Methods." *Communications in Soil Science and Plant Analysis*, 41(1), 22-31.

8

Estimation of Phosphorus and Potassium Cations in Plant Tissue

Sample Digestion

Dry ashing and wet oxidation are two widely adopted methods for releasing mineral elements from plant tissues. Dry ashing, typically conducted at temperatures between 550 and 600 °C, can lead to the loss of phosphorus (P) and potassium (K) through volatilization. This method is more time-consuming and has several drawbacks, such as the volatilization of sulfur (S) and chlorine (Cl), which can be mitigated by adding sodium carbonate (Na_2CO_3). Additionally, some phosphorus and micronutrients may become occluded during the process, making dry ashing less commonly used.

In contrast, wet oxidation employs oxidizing acids, such as a mixture of nitric acid and perchloric acid (HNO_3-$HClO_4$) or a tri-acid mixture of nitric acid, sulfuric acid, and perchloric acid (HNO_3-H_2SO_4-$HClO_4$). The use of perchloric acid ($HClO_4$) prevents the volatilization loss of potassium (K) and provides a clear solution, while sulfuric acid (H_2SO_4) aids in completing the oxidation. Upon heating, perchloric acid dissociates into nascent chlorine and oxygen, enhancing the oxidation efficiency at high temperatures. However, direct contact between perchloric acid and plant samples can lead to explosions and fires; thus, pre-digestion of samples is preferred.

Digestion with a HNO_3-$HClO_4$ mixture is often used instead of the tri-acid mixture, especially when sulfur (S) determination is also required in the same digest. The wet oxidation method is less time-consuming, easier, and more convenient compared to dry ashing.

TRI-ACID Digestion

Equipments and apparatus: Water bath, Hot plate

Reagent: Tri-acid mixture: Mix AR grade conc. HNO_3, H_2SO_4 and $HClO_4$ in 10:1:4 ratio and cool.

Procedure

1. Weigh 0.5 to 1.0 g of dried and processed plant sample to a 100/150 ml conical flask and add 5 ml of conc. HNO_3 to it.
2. Keep a glass funnel on the flask, place it on a water bath and heat at 100 °C for about 30 minutes and shift the flask to a hot plate and heat at 180-200 °C.
3. Continue boiling until near to dryness, but not drying completely. Cool and add 5 ml of the tri-acid mixture and heat at 180-200 °C.
4. Dense white fumes will evolve and continue digestion until the mixture is largely volatilized.
5. Remove the flasks when only moist, clear and white contents are left. The entire quantity of $HClO_4$ has volatilized by this stage.
6. Cool and add about 50 ml of distilled water or doubled distilled water if micronutrients are to be determined.
7. Filter into 100 ml flask, giving washings to make the volume to 100 ml.
8. The filtrate is ready to undergo further analysis.

DI-Acid Digestion

Equipments and apparatus: Hot plate

Reagent: Conc. HNO_3, 60% $HClO_4$ and approximately 2 N HCl

Procedure

1. Transfer 0.5 to 1.0 g of dried and processed plant sample in a 100/150 ml conical flask.
2. Add 10 ml of conc. HNO_3, place a funnel on the flask and keep for about 6-8 hours or overnight at a covered place/ chamber for pre-digestion.
3. After pre-digestion when the solid sample is no more visible, add 10 ml of conc. HNO_3 and 2-3 ml of $HClO_4$.
4. Keep on a hot plate in acid-proof digestion chamber having fume exhaust system and heat at about 100 °C for first one hour and then raise the temperature to about 200 °C.
5. Continue digestion until the contents become colorless and only white dense fumes appear.

6. Reduce the acid contents to about 2-3 ml by continuing heating at the same temperature. Do not allow to dry up.
7. Remove the flasks from hot plate, cool and add about 30 ml of distilled water.
8. Filter the solution through whatman no. 42 filter paper into a 100 ml volumetric flask.
9. Give 3-4 washings of 10-12 ml portions of distilled water and make the volume to 100 ml.

Phosphorus

Principle

Phosphorus can be determined using the methods based on molybdophosphoric blue colour developed by reduction of the heteropoly complex, or by vanadomolybdophosphoric yellow colour method. The development of yellow colour is due to substitution of oxyvanadium and oxymolydenum radicals for the PO_4 to give a heteropoly compound of the colour.

$$H_3PO_4 + 12\ H_2MoO_4 \rightarrow H_3P(Mo_3O_{10})_4 + 12\ H_2O$$

This method is suitable for P determination in plant extracts because the yellow colour developed is more stable than blue colour methods, no reductant is needed and no interference of other ions takes place even if present up to 1000 mg L^{-1} concentration.

Equipments and apparatus: Spectrophotometer or colorimeter, 50 ml volumetric flasks, pipettes, 1 L volumetric flasks, etc.

Reagents

1. Vanadomolybdate reagent: It is prepared by mixing two solutions

   Solution 1: Dissolve 25 g of ammonium molybdate $(NH_4)_6Mo_7O_{24}.4H_2O$ in 400 ml of warm distilled water and cool.

   Solution 2: Add slowly 1.25 g of ammonium metavandate to 300 ml of boiling water and cool. Then 250 ml of concentrated HNO_3 is added to it and allow it to cool.

   Pour the solution 2 into a one litre volumetric flask and add solution 1 to it. Mix properly and dilute to the mark with distilled water.

2. Standard P solution: Dissolve 0.2195 g of KH_2PO_4 and dilute to 1 L. This solution contains 50 ppm of P. Use this stock solution for preparation of standard curve for P.

Procedure

1. Take 10 ml of digested plant solution in a 50 ml volumetric flask.
2. Add 10 ml of nitric acid-molybdatevandatemixture, dilute the volume and mix thoroughly.
3. The colour develops fully within 30 minutes, which is stable for even 2 week to 2 months depending upon the concentration of P in plant tissue.
4. Read the intensity of yellow colour formed in spectrophotometer at a wavelength of 420 nm.
5. Run a blank (without P) simultaneously.
6. Pipette out 1.0, 1.5, 2.0, 2.5, 3.0, 4.0 and 5 ml of 50 ppm solution separately in 50 ml volumetric flask and develop colour in identical manner.
7. Prepare standard curve by plotting P concentrations on X-axis and per cent transmission/ colorimeter readings on Y-axis.

Calculation

$$\text{P in plant sample (ppm)} = \frac{\text{S-B}}{\text{A} \times \text{W}} \times \text{V}$$

% P in plant sample = ppm P in plant sample x 100/ 10^6

Where, S is µg P per 50 ml of colored complex made from an aliquot of sample digest as estimated by reference to the standard P graph.

B is µg P per 50 ml of colored complex made from an aliquot of blank digest.

V is total volume of the plant sample triacid digest in ml.

A is an aliquot of sample triacid digest in ml taken for the colour development.

W is the mass of plant sample in gram taken for the preparation of triacid digest.

Potassium

Potassium can also be determined from the same plant digest used for phosphorus by following standard procedures as employed in determination of K nutrient in soil. It can be determined by taking a suitable aliquot of the plant digest and inserting it to a flame photometer after proper dilution. For example, wheat grain digest can be taken up directly while straw samples are diluted 10 times.

9

Estimation of Secondary Nutrients and Micronutrient Cations in Plant Tissue

Sample Digestion

Dry ashing and wet oxidation are the two widely adopted methods for the release of mineral elements from plant tissues. Dry ashing is carried out usually at an ignition of 550 to 600 °C leads to loss of P and K by volatilization. Dry ashing being comparatively more time taking and also has a few drawbacks (such as S and Cl is lost by volatilization during ignition which can be prevented by adding Na_2CO_3; a part of P and micronutrients also get occluded) is hence occasionally adopted. On the other hand, wet oxidation employs oxidizing acids like HNO_3-$HClO_4$ di-acid or HNO_3-H_2SO_4-$HClO_4$ tri-acid mixture. The volatilization loss of K is prevented by the use of $HClO_4$ and provides a clear solution while H_2SO_4 helps completing oxidation. On heating $HClO_4$ dissociates into nascent chlorine and oxygen, increasing the oxidation efficiency at high temperature. Explosion and fire may occur if there is direct contact of $HClO_4$ with plant sample; hence the pre-digestion of samples is preferred. Digestion with HNO_3-$HClO_4$ instead of tri-acid mixture is also adopted specially when S is also to be determined in the same digest. The wet oxidation method being less time-consuming, easier and convenient is given below:

TRI-Acid Digestion

Equipments and apparatus: Water bath, Hot plate

Reagents: Tri-acid mixture: Mix AR grade conc. HNO_3, H_2SO_4 and $HClO_4$ in 10:1:4 ratio and cool.

Procedure

1. Weigh 0.5 to 1.0 g of dried and processed plant sample to a 100/150 ml conical flask and add 5 ml of conc. HNO_3 into it.
2. Keep a glass funnel on the flask, place it on a water bath and heat at 100 °C for about 30 minutes and shift the flask to a hot plate and heat at 180-200 °C.

3. Continue boiling until near to dryness, but not drying completely. Cool and add 5 ml of the tri-acid mixture and heat at 180-200 °C.
4. Dense white fumes will evolve and continue digestion until the mixture is largely volatilized.
5. Remove the flasks when only moist, clear and white contents are left. The entire quantity of $HClO_4$ has volatilized by this stage.
6. Cool and add about 50 ml of distilled water or doubled distilled water if micronutrients are to be determined.
7. Filter into 100 ml flask, giving washings to make the volume to 100 ml.
8. The filtrate is ready to undergo further analysis.

DI-Acid Digestion

Equipments and apparatus: Hot plate

Reagent: Conc. HNO_3, 60% $HClO_4$ and approx. 2 N HCl

Procedure

1. Transfer 0.5 to 1.0 g of dried and processed plant sample in a 100/150 ml conical flask.
2. Add 10 ml of conc. HNO_3, place a funnel on the flask and keep for about 6-8 hours or overnight at a covered place/ chamber for pre-digestion.
3. After pre-digestion when the solid sample is no more visible, add 10 ml of conc. HNO_3 and 2-3 ml of $HClO_4$.
4. Keep on a hot plate in acid-proof digestion chamber having fume exhaust system and heat at about 100 °C for first one hour and then raise the temperature to about 200 °C.
5. Continue digestion until the contents become colorless and only white dense fumes appear.
6. Reduce the acid contents to about 2-3 ml by continuing heating at the same temperature. Do not allow to dry up.
7. Remove the flasks from hot plate, cool and add about 30ml of distilled water.
8. Filter the solution through whatman No. 42 filter paper into a 100 ml volumetric flask.

9. Give 3-4 washings of 10-12 ml portions of distilled water and make the volume to 100 ml.

Calcium and Magnesium

Calcium and Magnesium can be determined in the di-acid digest of plant sample by using versene titration method or AAS. The element calcium can also be determined using a flame photometer, though the sensitivity is less than that for K and Na.

Sulphur

Wet oxidation based on tri-acid mixture includes H_2SO_4 and dry ashing leads to volatilization loss of S present in the organic combination, both of these techniques cannot be used for S determination in plant samples. Hence, HNO_3-$HClO_4$ is the appropriate digest to use for S extraction in plants. The S in the plant digest can be determined by turbidimetric method as described for soil sulphur.

Iron, Zinc, Manganese and Copper

The best and convenient method to determine the micronutrient cations in the di-acid digest of plant tissues is by using AAS as in case of soil analysis. Ortho phenanthroline method for Fe, Na-paraperiodate method for Mn and dithizone method for Zn and Cu can be used as alternative colorimetric methods.

Boron

For determination of B in plant tissue, following steps should be undergone:

1. Proceed for dry ashing with 0.5 g sample.
2. Extract the dry ash with 10 ml of 0.1 N HCl.
3. Filter or centrifuge the suspension to a clear state.
4. Pipette 1 ml of clear aliquot and proceed for azomethine-H method of B determination as described in case of soil.

Molybdenum

1. Take 1-10 g of sample in a platinum dish.
2. Perform dry ashing in an electric furnace at 500 °C.
3. Mix the ash with 2 g of anhydrous Na_2CO_3 at 1000 °C in the electric furnace, ensuring complete contact of the entire ash with the flux.

4. Cool the dish drop the cake into a 250 ml beaker by inverting the dish.
5. Measure the suspension in a cylinder and filter through Whatman No. 42 filter paper in a 250 ml beaker.
6. Measure the undiluted clear filtrate and use for Mo determination as described in soil analysis.
7. Calculate on the basis of the former volume.

10

Estimation of Electrical Conductivity in Soil

Objective

To determine the electrical conductivity (EC) of soil, which is an indicator of the soil's salinity and its ability to conduct electricity. This provides valuable information about the nutrient availability and potential toxicity to plants.

Materials Required

- Soil sample
- Distilled water
- Electrical conductivity meter (EC meter)
- Beakers (100 mL)
- Measuring cylinder (50 mL)
- Stirring rod
- Filter paper and funnel
- Mortar and pestle (for soil grinding, if necessary)

Principle

Electrical conductivity measures the ability of an aqueous solution to carry an electrical current, which depends on the presence of dissolved ions. In soils, salts like sodium chloride (NaCl), potassium nitrate (KNO_3), and calcium sulfate ($CaSO_4$) dissolve in water to form ions that contribute to the electrical conductivity. High EC values may indicate excessive salinity, which can affect plant growth.

Procedure

1. Soil Preparation

- Air-dry the soil sample if it is moist.
- Grind the soil gently using a mortar and pestle to break down larger aggregates.
- Sieve the soil through a 2 mm mesh to obtain a uniform sample.

2. Preparation of Soil Extract

- Take 20 g of the prepared soil sample and transfer it into a 100 mL beaker.
- Add 50 mL of distilled water to the soil sample (1:2.5 soil to water ratio).
- Stir the mixture thoroughly for 30 minutes using a stirring rod.
- Let the suspension settle for about 15-20 minutes.

3. Filtration

- Filter the soil-water suspension using filter paper and a funnel.
- Collect the filtrate in a clean beaker.

4. Measurement of Electrical Conductivity

- Calibrate the EC meter according to the manufacturer's instructions, using a standard conductivity solution.
- Rinse the EC meter probe with distilled water and gently wipe it with tissue paper.
- Immerse the EC meter probe in the soil extract (filtrate).
- Record the electrical conductivity reading in milliSiemens per centimeter (mS/cm).

5. Cleaning

- After the measurement, rinse the EC meter probe with distilled water and store it properly.

Calculation

- The EC value obtained from the meter is directly read in mS/cm.
- If necessary, adjust the reading based on the temperature of the solution, as EC is temperature-dependent.

Results

- Record the EC value of the soil sample.
- Compare the result with standard EC values to assess soil salinity levels.

Interpretation of Results

- Low EC (<0.2 mS/cm): Soil is low in salts, suitable for most crops.
- Moderate EC (0.2–0.8 mS/cm): Soil has moderate salinity; sensitive crops may be affected.
- High EC (0.8–2.0 mS/cm): Soil has high salinity; only salt-tolerant crops can grow.
- Very High EC (>2.0 mS/cm): Soil is highly saline, limiting the growth of most crops.

Precautions

- Ensure the soil sample is properly air-dried before testing.
- Calibrate the EC meter before each use for accurate results.
- Avoid contamination of the soil extract or EC meter probe.

References

Brady, N. C., & Weil, R. R. (2008). *The Nature and Properties of Soils* (14th ed.). Pearson Prentice Hall.

Gupta, P. K. (2000). *Methods in Environmental Analysis: Water, Soil, and Air*. Agrobios (India).

Rhoades, J. D. (1996). "Salinity: Electrical Conductivity and Total Dissolved Solids." In D.L. Sparks (Ed.), *Methods of Soil Analysis: Part 3 Chemical Methods*, Soil Science Society of America, pp. 417-435.

11

Determination of Soil pH

Objective

To determine the pH of a soil sample, which provides insight into the soil's acidity or alkalinity, influencing nutrient availability, microbial activity, and plant growth.

Materials Required

- Soil sample
- Distilled water
- pH meter or pH paper
- Beakers (100 mL)
- Measuring cylinder (50 mL)
- Stirring rod
- Filter paper and funnel (if needed)
- Mortar and pestle (for soil grinding, if necessary)

Principle

Soil pH measures the hydrogen ion concentration (H^+) in the soil. It affects the availability of nutrients and the activity of soil organisms. A pH value below 7 indicates acidic soil, while a value above 7 indicates alkaline soil. Most crops prefer a pH range between 6.0 and 7.5.

Procedure

1. Soil Preparation

- Air-dry the soil sample if moist.
- Grind the soil gently using a mortar and pestle to break down large aggregates.

- Sieve the soil through a 2 mm mesh to obtain a uniform sample.

2. Preparation of Soil Suspension

- Weigh 20 g of the prepared soil sample and transfer it into a 100 mL beaker.
- Add 50 mL of distilled water (1:2.5 soil to water ratio).
- Stir the mixture thoroughly for 30 minutes using a stirring rod.
- Let the soil suspension settle for about 15-20 minutes.

3. Measurement of Soil pH

- **If using a pH meter**
    - Calibrate the pH meter using standard buffer solutions (pH 4.0, 7.0, and 9.2) as per the manufacturer's instructions.
    - Rinse the pH meter probe with distilled water and gently blot it dry.
    - Immerse the pH probe in the soil suspension, ensuring it does not touch the sediment.
    - Wait for the reading to stabilize, then record the pH value.
- **If using pH paper**
    - Dip a strip of pH paper into the clear part of the soil suspension.
    - Compare the color change with the standard pH color chart provided with the pH paper.

4. Cleaning

- After measurement, rinse the pH meter probe with distilled water and store it as per the instructions.

Results

- Record the pH value of the soil sample.

Interpretation of Results

- Strongly acidic (<5.0): Unsuitable for most crops; lime application may be necessary.
- Moderately acidic (5.0–6.0): Suitable for acid-loving plants; limited availability of certain nutrients.

- Slightly acidic (6.0–6.5): Ideal for most crops.
- Neutral (6.5–7.5): Optimal for a wide range of crops.
- Slightly alkaline (7.5–8.5): Some nutrients may become less available, especially phosphorus.
- Strongly alkaline (>8.5): Nutrient availability decreases; may require sulfur application or other amendments.

Precautions

- Ensure that the soil sample is representative of the field.
- Always calibrate the pH meter before use for accurate results.
- Avoid touching the pH meter probe directly to soil particles, as it can damage the sensor.

References

Brady, N. C., & Weil, R. R. (2008). The *Nature and Properties of Soils (1*4th ed.). Pearson Prentice Hall.

Gupta, P. K. (2000). Methods in Environmental *Analysis: Water, Soil, and Air. Agrobios (India). McLean, E. O. (1982).* "Soil pH and Lime Requirement." In Methods of Soil Analysis Part 2: *Chemical and Microbiological Properties, Soil Science* Society of America, pp. 199-224.

Rayment, G. E., & Lyons, *D. J. (2010). Soil Chemical Meth*ods: Australasia. CSIRO Publishing.

12

Estimation of Soil Organic Carbon

The Walkley-Black method is a widely used chemical procedure to estimate soil organic carbon (SOC). It involves the oxidation of organic carbon by potassium dichromate in the presence of sulfuric acid, followed by titration to determine the amount of unreacted dichromate. Here is a detailed step-by-step guide:

Materials Required

- Soil sample (air-dried and sieved through a 2 mm sieve)
- Potassium dichromate solution (1 N)
- Concentrated sulfuric acid (H_2SO_4)
- Ferrous ammonium sulfate solution (0.5 N)
- Orthophosphoric acid (H_3PO_4) (optional)
- Diphenylamine indicator or N-phenylanthranilic acid (indicator)
- Distilled water
- Burette, pipette, and conical flasks
- Heating mantle or hot plate

Procedure

1. Sample Preparation

- Air-dry the soil sample and sieve it through a 2 mm sieve to remove large particles and organic debris.

2. Weighing the Soil

- Accurately weigh 0.5 to 1.0 g of the sieved soil sample. The exact amount depends on the expected organic carbon content; generally, 1 g is used for soils with low organic carbon content, and 0.5 g for soils with high organic carbon content.

3. Addition of Potassium Dichromate

- Transfer the weighed soil sample into a 250 mL conical flask.
- Add 10 mL of 1 N potassium dichromate solution to the soil in the flask using a pipette.

4. Addition of Sulfuric Acid

- Carefully add 20 mL of concentrated sulfuric acid to the flask containing the soil and dichromate solution. Add the acid slowly, swirling the flask gently to ensure thorough mixing.
- This step oxidizes the organic carbon in the soil. The mixture should turn dark green if carbon is present.

5. Heating (Optional)

- Heat the mixture for 5-10 minutes at 130-150°C on a heating mantle or hot plate. Heating ensures complete oxidation of the organic carbon. This step is optional but recommended for high organic matter soils.

6. Cooling the Mixture

- Allow the mixture to cool to room temperature. This may take around 30 minutes.

7. Dilution

- After cooling, add 200 mL of distilled water to dilute the reaction mixture. If the solution is still hot, add water slowly to prevent splashing.

8. Addition of Indicator

- Add 5-10 drops of the diphenylamine indicator (or N-phenylanthranilic acid). The indicator will help visualize the endpoint of the titration by changing the color from purple-blue to green.

9. Titration with Ferrous Ammonium Sulfate

- Titrate the mixture with 0.5 N ferrous ammonium sulfate solution until the color changes from purple-blue to green, indicating the endpoint.
- Record the volume of ferrous ammonium sulfate used.

10. Blank Titration

- Perform a blank titration without soil using the same amounts of potassium dichromate, sulfuric acid, and water to standardize the results.
- Record the volume of ferrous ammonium sulfate used for the blank.

Calculations

1. Determine the Amount of Potassium Dichromate Reacted

- Calculate the difference in volume of ferrous ammonium sulfate used between the blank and the soil sample titration.

2. Calculate the Organic Carbon Content

- Use the formula to calculate the organic carbon content:

$$\text{Organic carbon in soil (\%)} = \frac{10\,(B\text{-}S)}{B} \times 0.003 \times \frac{100}{\text{Weight of sample (g)}}$$

Where, B is titrated value (ml) of Blank sample

S is titrated value (ml) of Test sample

Low Organic Carbon Content: The solution may appear lighter blue.

High Organic Carbon Content: The solution may appear darker blue or green.

References

Nelson, D.W., & Sommers, L.E. (1982). Total Carbon, Organic Carbon, and Organic Matter. In A. L. Page et al. (Eds.), Methods of Soil Analysis: Part 2. Chemical and Microbiological Properties (2nd ed., pp. 539-579). American Society of Agronomy.

Soil Science Society of America (2008). Soil Organic Carbon Storage and Its Environmental Implications. In J.D. Hill, C. E. K. Tsai, & R. M. Gephart (Eds.), Soil Organic Carbon and Soil Health (pp. 151-165). Soil Science Society of America.

Walkley, A., & Black, I.A. (1934). An Examination of the Degtjareff Method for Determining Soil Organic Matter, and a Proposed Modification of the Chromic Acid Titration Method. Soil Science, 37(1), 29-38.

13

Determination of Chlorophyll-A, Chlorophyll-B, and Total Chlorophyll Content of Leaves Based on Fresh Weight, Dry Weight and Leaf Area

Chlorophyll content serves as a vital indicator of plant health and photosynthetic efficiency, with higher levels reflecting robust photosynthesis and overall plant vigor, while lower levels may signal nutrient deficiencies, diseases, or environmental stresses. Assessing chlorophyll content helps evaluate plant productivity, as chlorophyll is essential for absorbing light and converting solar energy into chemical energy. Additionally, the chlorophyll-a to chlorophyll-b ratio provides insights into how plants adapt to various light conditions, revealing their light absorption efficiency and ability to cope with environmental changes. Measuring chlorophyll on a fresh weight, dry weight, and leaf area basis allows researchers and agronomists to gauge the effectiveness of agricultural practices such as fertilization, irrigation, and crop management strategies. It also aids in monitoring the impact of stress factors like drought, salinity, pollution, or pest attacks, which is crucial for developing strategies to enhance crop resilience.

Reagents: 80% acetone: - 80 ml acetone + 20 ml water = 100 ml

Procedure for Chlorophyll Extraction from Leaves

1. **Sample Collection**: Collect fresh, healthy leaves from the plant to be analyzed. Ensure that the leaves are free from dust, pests, and diseases.
2. **Preparation of Leaf Samples**: Rinse the leaves thoroughly with distilled water to remove any surface contaminants. Pat them dry with a clean paper towel. Weigh an exact amount (usually around 0.1-0.5 grams) of fresh leaf tissue using an analytical balance. Record the fresh weight accurately.
3. **Homogenization**: Cut the leaf samples into small pieces and place them in a mortar. Add 10-20 mL of 80% acetone or ethanol (depending on the

chosen solvent) to the mortar. Grind the leaves thoroughly with a pestle until a uniform paste is obtained, ensuring maximum extraction of the pigments.

4. **Filtration**: Transfer the homogenized mixture into a centrifuge tube or through a funnel lined with filter paper. If using a centrifuge, centrifuge the mixture at 4,000-5,000 RPM for 5-10 minutes to separate the chlorophyll-containing solution from the leaf debris. If filtering, collect the filtrate in a clean container.

5. **Volume Adjustment**: Transfer the supernatant (chlorophyll extract) into a clean volumetric flask. Adjust the final volume to a known value (e.g., 25 or 50 mL) with the same solvent used for extraction (80% acetone or ethanol). Ensure thorough mixing.

6. **Spectrophotometric Measurement**: Pour a portion of the chlorophyll extract into a clean cuvette. Measure the absorbance of the solution at specific wavelengths using a spectrophotometer. Typically, readings are taken at 663 nm for chlorophyll-a and 645 nm for chlorophyll-b. Calibrate the spectrophotometer using the pure solvent as a blank.

7. **Calculation of Chlorophyll Content**: Use the absorbance values obtained to calculate the concentrations of chlorophyll-a, chlorophyll-b, and total chlorophyll in the leaf extract using the appropriate formulas:

$$\text{Chlorophyll-a (mg/g)} = \frac{12.7 \times A_{663} - 2.69 \times A_{645}}{\text{Fresh weight of leaf sample}}$$

$$\text{Chlorophyll-b (mg/g)} = \frac{22.9 \times A_{645} - 4.68 \times A_{663}}{\text{Fresh weight of leaf sample}}$$

$$\text{Total Chlorophyll (mg/g)} = \frac{20.2 \times A_{645} + 8.02 \times A_{663}}{\text{Fresh weight of leaf sample}}$$

Where A_{663} and A_{645} are the absorbance values at 663 nm and 645 nm, respectively.

8. **Repeat and Average**: Repeat the procedure for at least three replicates to ensure accuracy. Calculate the average chlorophyll content based on the replicates.

Precautions

- Ensure that the leaf samples are fresh and healthy, free from any signs of disease or physical damage, to obtain accurate chlorophyll content.

- Perform the extraction and analysis in dim light or under green light conditions, as chlorophyll is sensitive to light and can degrade rapidly upon exposure.
- Use clean glassware, cuvettes, and instruments throughout the experiment to avoid contamination that could affect the absorbance readings.
- Ensure that the acetone or ethanol used is of the correct concentration (typically 80%) to maximize chlorophyll extraction efficiency.
- Always calibrate the spectrophotometer with the solvent blank before taking measurements to obtain accurate absorbance values.
- Perform all steps promptly to prevent chlorophyll degradation, which can occur due to prolonged exposure to air, light, or heat.
- Accurately weigh the leaf samples and measure the volumes of solvents to ensure precise chlorophyll quantification.
- Handle solvents like acetone or ethanol with care, using gloves and working in a well-ventilated area to avoid inhalation or skin contact.

References

Arnon, D. I. (1949). "Copper Enzymes in Isolated Chloroplasts: Polyphenol oxidase in Beta vulgaris." *Plant Physiology*, 24(1), 1-15.

Inskeep, W. P., & Bloom, P. R. (1985). "Extinction Coefficients of Chlorophyll a and b in N, N-Dimethylformamide and 80% Acetone." *Plant Physiology*, 77(2), 483-485.

Lichtenthaler, H. K., & Wellburn, A. R. (1983). "Determinations of Total Carotenoids and Chlorophylls a and b of Leaf Extracts in Different Solvents." *Biochemical Society Transactions,* 11(5), 591-592.

Porra, R. J., Thompson, W. A., & Kriedemann, P. E. (1989). "Determination of Accurate Extinction Coefficients and Simultaneous Equations for Assaying Chlorophylls A and B Extracted with Four Different Solvents: Verification of the Concentration of Chlorophyll Standards by Atomic Absorption Spectroscopy." *Biochimica et Biophysica Acta (BBA) - Bioenergetics,* 975(3), 384-394.

Sadasivam, S. and Manickam, A. (1992). *Biochemical Methods for Agricultural Sciences.* p.184, Wiley Eastern Limited.

14

Determination of Carotenoid Content of Leaves

Introduction

Carotenoids are pigments found in plants that contribute to photosynthesis and provide various health benefits. Measuring carotenoid content in leaves can help assess plant health, productivity, and the effects of environmental conditions. The determination of carotenoids typically involves extraction followed by spectrophotometric analysis.

Materials and Equipments

- Fresh leaf samples
- Acetone, hexane, or a mixture of acetone and hexane (for extraction)
- Mortar and pestle or homogenizer
- Centrifuge and centrifuge tubes
- Spectrophotometer
- Volumetric flasks and pipettes
- Analytical balance

Procedure

1. Sample Preparation

- Collect fresh, healthy leaves and rinse them with distilled water to remove any surface contaminants.
- Dry the leaves thoroughly with a paper towel and weigh an exact amount (typically 0.1-0.5 grams) using an analytical balance.

2. Extraction

- Cut the leaves into small pieces and grind them in a mortar with 10-20 mL of an appropriate solvent (acetone, hexane, or a mixture of acetone and hexane). Ensure the grinding is thorough to maximize pigment extraction.

- Transfer the homogenized mixture into a centrifuge tube or a clean container. If using a centrifuge, centrifuge at 4,000-5,000 RPM for 5-10 minutes to separate the liquid extract from the solid leaf debris. Alternatively, filter the mixture through a funnel lined with filter paper.

3. Preparation of Extract

- Transfer the supernatant (carotenoid extract) into a clean volumetric flask. Adjust the final volume to a known value (e.g., 25 or 50 mL) with the same solvent used for extraction. Mix thoroughly.

4. Spectrophotometric Analysis

- Use a spectrophotometer to measure the absorbance of the carotenoid extract. Carotenoids typically absorb light at wavelengths between 400 nm and 480 nm.
- Measure the absorbance at specific wavelengths, such as 450 nm and 480 nm, which are commonly used for carotenoid analysis.

5. Calculation of Carotenoid Content

- Calculate the carotenoid content using the following formula, which uses the absorbance values and the concentration of the extract:

$$\text{Carotenoid content} = \left(\frac{\text{mg}}{\text{g}}\right) = \frac{A \times V \times F}{W \times L}$$

Where:

- A = Absorbance at the specific wavelength
- V = Volume of the extract (in mL)
- F = Dilution factor (if any)
- W = Weight of the leaf sample (in grams)
- L = Path length of the cuvette (in cm, usually 1 cm)

Note: Alternatively, use specific formulas and extinction coefficients provided in the literature for more accurate carotenoid quantification.

6. Repeat and Average

- Perform the procedure in triplicate or more to ensure accuracy and calculate the average carotenoid content.

Points to Remember

- Ensure that the leaf samples are fresh and free from signs of damage or decay, as deteriorated samples can affect carotenoid content and accuracy of results.
- Minimize exposure of leaf samples to light and heat during the extraction process, as carotenoids are sensitive to degradation from light and temperature.
- Thoroughly clean all glassware and tools with suitable cleaning agents and rinse them with distilled water before use to avoid contamination.
- Perform all extraction and analysis steps promptly to prevent oxidation of carotenoids. Use antioxidants or work in an inert atmosphere if necessary.
- Choose appropriate solvents for carotenoid extraction (such as acetone, hexane, or a mixture of acetone and hexane) and ensure they are of high purity to avoid interference.
- Grind the leaf samples thoroughly and ensure complete extraction of carotenoids to get accurate results. Incomplete extraction can lead to lower measured carotenoid content.
- When measuring absorbance with a spectrophotometer, ensure that the cuvette is placed correctly and at the same height as the reference cell to avoid parallax errors.
- Calibrate the spectrophotometer with the appropriate blank before measuring the carotenoid extract to ensure accurate absorbance readings.
- Perform all steps under subdued light or use green safety lighting to prevent carotenoid degradation due to exposure to visible light.
- Carry out the extraction and spectrophotometric analysis at a consistent temperature to ensure that variations do not affect the carotenoid content measurement.

References

Britton, G., Liaaen-Jensen, S., & Pfander, H. (2004). *Carotenoids: Volume 1A - Pigments of Plants and Algae*. Birkhäuser Basel.

Lichtenthaler, H. K., & Buschmann, C. (2001). "Chlorophylls and Carotenoids: Measurement and Characterization by UV-VIS Spectroscopy." In *Current Protocols in Food Analytical Chemistry* (pp. F4.3.1-F4.3.8). Wiley.

Wellburn, A. R. (1994). "The Spectral Determination of Chlorophylls a and b, as Well as Total Carotenoids, Using Various Solvents with Spectrophotometers of Different Resolution." *Journal of Plant Physiology*, 144(3), 307-313.

15

Determination of Leaf Relative Water Content

Leaf Relative Water Content (RWC) is a key indicator of plant water status and is used to assess water stress, physiological health, and the efficiency of water use in plants. It reflects the amount of water in the leaf relative to its maximum water capacity and is a useful measure in plant physiology and stress studies.

Materials and Equipment

- Fresh leaf samples
- Analytical balance
- Oven or drying equipment
- Desiccator
- Caliper or ruler
- Distilled water
- Petri dishes or similar containers
- Weighing boats or paper

Procedure

1. Sample Collection

- Collect fresh, healthy leaves from the plant, ensuring they are free from damage or disease. The leaves should be collected at the same time of day to minimize diurnal variations in water content.

2. Fresh Weight Measurement

- Weigh the fresh leaf samples accurately using an analytical balance. Record the fresh weight (W_{fresh}).

3. Turgid Weight Measurement

- Immerse the fresh leaf samples in distilled water for 4-6 hours or until they reach full turgidity. Ensure that the leaves are fully submerged and not folded or crumpled.
- After the immersion period, gently blot the leaves with a paper towel to remove excess surface water, then weigh them again. Record the turgid weight (W_{turgid}).

4. Dry Weight Measurement

- Dry the turgid leaves in an oven at a temperature of 70-80°C for 24-48 hours, or until they reach a constant weight. This ensures that all moisture is removed.
- After drying, cool the leaves in a desiccator and weigh them. Record the dry weight (W_{dry}).

5. Calculate Relative Water Content (RWC)

$$RWC\ (\%) = \frac{W_{fresh} - W_{dry}}{W_{turgid} - W_{dry}} \times 100$$

Where: W_{fresh} = Fresh weight of the leaf (g)

W_{turgid} = Turgid weight of the leaf (g)

W_{dry} = Dry weight of the leaf (g)

6. Repeat Measurements

- Perform the procedure with multiple leaf samples to ensure accuracy and calculate the average RWC.

Precautions

1. **Use Uniform Leaf Samples**: Ensure that leaf samples are of similar size and age to obtain consistent and comparable results.
2. **Minimize Water Loss**: Handle the leaf samples carefully to prevent water loss before measurement. Work quickly to avoid desiccation.
3. **Accurate Weighing**: Use an analytical balance for precise measurements of fresh, turgid, and dry weights to ensure accurate RWC calculations.

4. **Proper Drying**: Dry the leaves completely to a constant weight to avoid errors in the calculation of dry weight.

5. **Prevent Contamination**: Use clean equipment and containers to avoid contamination that could affect weight measurements.

6. **Consistent Immersion Time**: Immerse leaves for a consistent period to ensure uniform turgidity across samples.

7. **Avoid Excessive Blotting**: Gently blot the turgid leaves to remove surface water without squeezing or damaging the leaf tissue.

References

Bartlett, M. K., & Cernusak, L. A. (2019). "Measuring the Water Content of Leaves and Its Effect on Photosynthesis." *Plant Methods,* 15, 79.

Gitelson, A. A., & Merzlyak, M. N. (1998). "Signature Analysis of Leaf Reflectance Spectra for Estimating Chlorophyll Content." *Journal of Plant Physiology,* 154(5), 821-829.

Liu, X., & Lu, X. (2007). "Determination of Relative Water Content in Plant Leaves." *Plant Physiology,* 43(4), 556-559.

Turner, N. C. (1988). "Measurement of Plant Water Status by the Pressure Chamber Technique." *Irrigation Science*, 9(3), 145-154.

16

General Considerations of Analytical Determination

Analytical Reagents

Chemical reagents are supplied in different grades and each grade has a distinct purpose and range of uses. The purest grade is analytical reagent (AR), the second is laboratory reagent (LR), the third is guaranteed reagent (GR) and fourth is technical grade. Second and third form of reagents have a lot of impurities. Therefore, for the determination of micronutrients, AR grade reagents should be used.

Distilled Water

Distilled water is always used in chemical analysis. The quality of distilled water varies from single distilled water to double or triple distilled water depending upon the requirement of analytical technique(s) e.g. double distilled water (glass distilled) is always recommended for micro nutrient and heavy-metal analysis.

Filter Paper

Several types of filter papers are available in the market depending on their ash content, porosity and elemental composition. The commonly used filter papers are Whatman, Munktells, Schleicher and Schuell. These filter papers are available in different number(s) ranging from No.1 to 60. The pore size decreases with their increasing numbers.

Solute

The minor component in a solution, dissolved in the solvent.

Solvent

A solvent is the component of a solution that is present in the greatest amount. It is the substance in which the solute is dissolved. Examples: The solvent for seawater is water.

Solution

The dispersion of a substance in molecular or ionic form throughout the medium of another is known as solution. A solution contains both solute and solvent. True solution is homogenous mixture of solute and solvent although they differ in their molecular structure. Size of the solute is less than 0.001 μm in diameter.

Acid

An acid is a substance that increases the concentration of hydrogen ions (H^+) when dissolved in water. $HA \leftrightarrow H^{++} A^-$

Base

A base is a substance that increases the concentration of hydroxyl (OH^-) ion when dissolved in water.

pH

The pH of a solution expresses the concentration of hydrogen (H^+) ion in the solution. It is calculated as the negative logarithm of hydrogen ion concentration. Solutions with pH below 7 are increasingly acidic as pH value decreases. Solutions with pH values above 7 are increasingly basic as pH value increases. Since normal water has a pH value of 7, it is placed in the middle of the scale and considered neutral.

Pure water has almost the same concentration of hydrogen ions as hydroxyl ions since there is almost no dissociation. Even so, the concentration of hydroxyl ions is 1.0×10^7 moles/liter more than that of hydrogen ions i.e. pure water is negligibly negatively ionized. Thus, the pH of pure water is

$$pH = -Log_{10}(1.0\times10^7)$$

$$= -7\times -Log_{10} 10$$

$$= -7\times -1 (because\ Log_{10}=1)$$

$$= 7.0$$

Concentration

Concentration refers to the amount of a substance per defined space. Another definition is that concentration is the ratio of solute in a solution to either solvent or total solution. Concentration usually is expressed in terms of mass per unit volume.

Standard Solution

A standard solution is a solution containing a precisely known concentration of an element or a substance. A known weight of solute is dissolved to make a specific volume.

Saturated Solution

A saturated solution is a chemical solution containing the maximum concentration of a solute dissolved in the solvent. The additional solute will not dissolve in a saturated solution.

Unsaturated Solution

An unsaturated solution is a chemical solution in which the solute concentration is lower than its equilibrium solubility.

Super Saturated Solution

Supersaturation is a solution that contains more of the dissolved material than could be dissolved by the solvent under normal circumstances.

Molar Solution

Molar solution is one in which the gram molecular weight of substance is dissolved in a solvent, whose volume is adjusted to one litre. For example: 342 g of sucrose (i.e. 1gram molecular weight) is dissolved in some water (500 ml) and its volume is adjusted to exact 1 litre. Resultant solution is called *molar solution* of sucrose and its strength is called molarity.

Molal Solution

Molal solution is one in which the gram molecular weight of substance is dissolved in one litre of solvent. Its volume exceeds one litre ie. of molar solution. Hence it is more diluted than molar solution. 342 g of sucrose dissolved in one litre of water yields molal solution of sucrose and its strength is called molality.

Normal Solution

A gram equivalent weight of a substance dissolved in one lire yields normal solution and its strength is called normality.

Parts per million solution-(ppm=mg/litre) 1 mg of a substance when dissolved in one litre of solvent, yields 1 ppm solution i.e. particular weight in mg of a substance dissolved in one litre of solvent, yields ppm solution of that same particular strength.

Percent Solution

1. V/V- The particular volume of a particular liquid dissolved in another liquid whose volume is adjusted to 100ml, yields percentage solution. If the solute is 2ml then the strength of solution will be 2%.

2. W/V- 2g of a substance dissolved in water to make a final volume of 100 ml yields 2%.

Reference

Rana, D.S. (2002). Yield and yield attributes, nutrients uptake, nitrogen-use efficiency and economics of oleiferous brassicas as influenced by time of sowing and fertility levels. *Indian J. Agric. Sci.* 72(9):519 to 524.

17

Preparation and Standardization of Buffer Solutions for Laboratory Applications

Buffers

Bronsted and Lowry defined acids as substances which are able to donate protons, and bases as substances which accept protons.

$$BH \longrightarrow B^- + H^+$$

In the above example, BH is an acid because it donates proton and B^- is an anion liberated by the deprotonation of the acid. B^- behaves like a base, so it is called conjugate base.

Acids can be classified into strong acids and weak acids.

1. **Strong acids** get dissociated almost completely, e.g., hydrochloric acid, sulphuric acid. This is because the conjugate bases of these acids are very weak (have less affinity for the proton).

2. **Weak acids** get dissociated partially, e.g., acetic acid, carbonic acid. This happens because the conjugate bases of these acids are strong (have greater affinity for proton). Since the dissociation of the weak acids is partial, the equilibrium constant for the dissociation reaction of the weak acid (BH) can be written as follows:

$$BH \longrightarrow B^- + H^+$$

$$Ka = \frac{[B^-]\,[H^+]}{[BH]}$$

The equilibrium constants for ionization reactions are commonly called **ionization or dissociation constant (Ka).** The above equation can be rearranged as:

$$[H^+] = \frac{Ka \times [BH]}{[B^-]}$$

By multiplying the above equation by –1 and taking logarithm of both sides, the following expression can be derived:

$$-[H^+] = -\left[\frac{Ka \times [BH]}{[B^-]}\right]$$

$$-\log_{10}[H^+] = -\log_{10} Ka - \log_{10}\frac{[BH]}{[B^-]}$$

$$-\log_{10}[H^+] \text{ is pH}$$

As the hydrogen ion concentration increases, the pH of the solution decreases. As the hydrogen ion concentration decreases, pH will increase. Hydrogen ion concentration and pH are reciprocally related.

$$pH = pKa + \log_{10}\frac{[B^-]}{[BH]}$$

$$pH = pKa + \log_{10}\frac{[\text{Conjugate base}]}{[\text{Acid}]}$$

CH_3COOH + NaCl

This expression is called **Henderson-Hasselbalch equation**. If the conjugate base and acid concentration is the same, then **pH = pKa**. The value of pKa is lower for strong acids and higher for weak acids.

Buffers: - A buffer solution is one which resist change in its pH when small amount of acid or base is added to it. Buffer solutions are composed of a weak acid (the proton donor) and its conjugate base (the proton acceptor). Buffering results from two reversible reaction equilibria in a solution wherein the concentration of proton donor and its conjugate proton acceptor are equal.

Most simple buffers work effectively in the pH scale of pKa ± 1.0.

Mechanism of Buffer Action

The most common types of buffers are mixtures of weak acids and salts of their conjugate bases, for example, acetic acid/sodium acetate. When a strong acid is added, protons are scavenged by the salt component of the buffer system. Similarly, when an alkali is added, acid component will get deprotonated and the alkali combines with the proton to form water. Acetate buffer is made up of acetic acid and sodium acetate (CH_3COOH / CH_3COONa).

(a) When acid like HCl is added to the acetate buffer system, CH_3COONa gets converted to CH_3COO^-. Acetate combines with the protons released by the strong acids to give acetic acid, which is a weak acid, and the change in pH is very small.

(b) When a strong alkali like NaOH is added, OH^- combines with the H^+ released by the CH_3COOH to form water. Na^+ combines with acetate to form sodium acetate.

$$NaOH \longrightarrow Na^+ + OH^-$$

$$CH_3COOH \longrightarrow CH_3COO^- + H^-$$

$$CH_3COO^- \xrightarrow{Na^+} CH_3COONa \qquad H^- \xrightarrow{OH^-} H_2O$$

$$CH_3COONa + H_2O$$

Buffering Capacity

Buffer capacity is a term used to describe the ability of a given buffer to resist changes in pH on addition of acid or base. A buffer capacity of 1 is when 1 mol of acid or alkali is added to 1 litre of buffer and pH changes by 1 unit.

Buffering capacity depends upon the following factors:

1. The concentration of the acid and base component of the buffer

As the concentration of acid and base component of the buffer increases, buffering capacity of the buffer also increases.

2. The pH of the Buffer

Buffer can act best at pH = pKa, and its buffering range is about one pH unit above or below the pKa value.

Preparation of some common Buffers

M Glycine-HCl Buffer; pH range 2.2 to 3.6

(a) 0.1 M Glycine: 7.5 g/l (M.W.: 75.0)

(b) 0.1 M Hydrochloric acid

Mix 50 ml of glycine and indicated volume of hydrochloric acid. Mix and adjust the final volume to 100 ml with deionized water. Adjust the final pH using a sensitive pH meter.

ml of HCl	44.0	32.4	24.2	16.8	11.4	8.2	6.4	5.0
pH	2.2	2.4	2.6	2.8	3.0	3.2	3.4	3.6

M Hydrochloric Acid-Potassium Chloride Buffer (HCl-KCl); pH Range 1.0 to 2.2

(a) 0.1 M Potassium chloride: 7.45 g/l (M.W.: 74.5)

(b) 0.1 M Hydrochloric acid

Mix 50 ml of potassium chloride and indicated volume of hydrochloric acid. Mix and adjust the final volume to 100 ml with deionized water. Adjust the final pH using a sensitive pH meter.

ml of HCl	97.0	64.5	41.5	26.3	16.6	10.6	6.7
pH	1.0	1.2	1.4	1.6	1.8	2.0	2.2

3. M Citrate Buffer; pH range 3.0 to 6.2

(a) 0.1 M Citric acid: 19.21 g/l (M.W.: 192.1)

(b) 0.1 M Sodium citrate dihydrate: 29.4 g/l (M.W.: 294.0)

Mix citric acid and sodium citrate solutions in the proportions indicated and adjust the final volume to 100 ml with deionized water. Adjust the final pH using a sensitive pH meter. The use of pentahydrate salt of sodium citrate is not recommended.

ml of Citric acid	46.5	40.0	35.0	31.5	25.5	20.5	16.0	11.8	7.2
ml of Sodium citrate	3.5	10.0	15.0	18.5	24.5	29.5	34.0	38.2	42.8
pH	3.0	3.4	3.8	4.2	4.6	5.0	5.4	5.8	6.2

4. M Acetate Buffer; pH range 3.6 to 5.6

(a) 0.1 M Acetic acid (5.8 ml made to 1000 ml)

(b) 0.1 M Sodium acetate; 8.2 g/l (anhydrous; M.W. 82.0) or 13.6 g/l(trihydrate; M.W. 136.0)

Mix acetic acid and sodium acetate solutions in the proportions indicated and adjust the final volume to 100 ml with deionized water. Adjust the final pH using a sensitive pH meter.

ml of Acetic acid	46.3	41.0	30.5	20.0	14.8	10.5	4.8
ml of Sodium acetate	3.7	9.0	19.5	30.0	35.2	39.5	45.2
pH	3.6	4.0	4.4	4.8	5.0	5.2	5.6

5. M Citrate-Phosphate Buffer; pH range 2.6 to 7.0

(a) 0.1 M Citric acid; 19.21 g/l (M.W. 192.1)

(b) 0.2 M Dibasic sodium phosphate; 35.6 g/l (dihydrate; M.W. 178.0) or 53.6 g/l heptahydrate; M.W. 268.0)

Mix citric acid and sodium phosphate solutions in the proportions indicated and adjust the final volume to 100 ml with deionized water. Adjust the final pH using a sensitive pH meter.

ml of Citric acid	44.6	39.8	35.9	32.3	29.4	26.7	24.3	22.2	19.7	16.9	13.6	6.5
ml of Sodium phosphate	5.4	10.2	14.1	17.7	20.6	23.3	25.7	27.8	30.3	33.1	36.4	43.6
pH	2.6	3.0	3.4	3.8	4.2	4.6	5.0	5.4	5.8	6.2	6.6	7.0

6. Phosphate Buffer; pH range 5.8 to 8.0

(a) 0.1 M Sodium phosphate monobasic; 13.8 g/l (monohydrate, M.W. 138.0)

(b) 0.1 M Sodium phosphate dibasic; 26.8 g/l (heptahydrate, M.W. 268.0)

Mix sodium phosphate monobasic and dibasic solutions in the proportions indicated and adjust the final volume to 200 ml with deionized water. Adjustthe final pH using a sensitive pH meter.

ml of Sodium phosphate, Mono-basic	92.0	81.5	73.5	62.5	51.0	39.0	28.0	19.0	13.0	8.5	5.3
ml of Sodium phosphate, Dibasic	8.0	18.5	26.5	37.5	49.0	61.0	72.0	81.0	87.0	91.5	94.7
pH	5.8	6.2	6.4	6.6	6.8	7.0	7.2	7.4	7.6	7.8	8.0

7. Tris-HCl Buffer, pH range 7.2 to 9.0

(a) 0.1 M Tris (hydroxymethyl) aminomethane; 12.1 g/l (M.W.: 121.0)

(b) 0.1 M Hydrochloric acid

Mix 50 ml of Tris(hydroxymethyl)aminomethane and indicated volume of hydrochloric acid and adjust the final volume to 200 ml with deionized water. Adjust the final pH using a sensitive pH meter.

ml of HCl	44.2	41.4	38.4	32.5	21.9	12.2	5.0

pH	7.2	7.4	7.6	7.8	8.2	8.6	9.0

8. Carbonate-Bicarbonate Buffer, pH range 9.2 to 10.6

(a) 0.1 M Sodium carbonate (anhydrous), 10.6 g/l (M.W.: 106.0)

(b) 0.1 M Sodium bicarbonate, 8.4 g/l (M.W.: 84.0)

Mix sodium carbonate and sodium bicarbonate solutions in the proportions indicated and adjust the final volume to 200 ml with deionized water. Adjust the final pH usinga sensitive pH meter.

ml of Sodium carbonate	4.0	9.5	16.0	22.0	27.5	33.0	38.5	42.5
ml of Sodium bicarbonate	46.0	40.5	34.0	28.0	22.5	17.0	11.5	7.5
pH	9.2	9.4	9.6	9.8	10.0	10.2	10.4	10.6

18

General Precautions for Volumetric and Gravimetric Analysis

Volumetric Analysis Precautions

1. **Use Clean Glassware:** Ensure all glassware, such as burettes, pipettes, and volumetric flasks, is thoroughly cleaned and rinsed with distilled water to avoid contamination and ensure accurate measurements.
2. **Clean Glassware Properly:** Before use, all glass apparatus should be thoroughly cleaned with a cleansing mixture of potassium dichromate ($K_2Cr_2O_7$) and concentrated sulfuric acid (H_2SO_4) to remove any residual contaminants. After cleaning, rinse the glassware thoroughly with distilled water to ensure no traces of the cleansing mixture remain.
3. **Proper Calibration:** Calibrate all measuring instruments, including burettes, pipettes, and balances, before use to maintain accuracy in measurements.
4. **Avoid Parallax Error:** When reading the meniscus level in a burette or volumetric flask, ensure the eye is at the same level as the meniscus to prevent parallax error.
5. **Use Correct Indicators:** Choose the appropriate indicator for the titration based on the type of reaction and the pH range of the endpoint to ensure precise determination of the endpoint.
6. **Control Temperature:** Perform titrations at a consistent temperature, preferably at room temperature, as temperature variations can affect the volume measurements and reaction rates.
7. **Add Reagents Slowly:** Add titrants slowly and dropwise, especially near the endpoint, to avoid overshooting and ensure an accurate determination of the endpoint.
8. **Mix Solutions Thoroughly:** Swirl the flask gently and continuously during titration to ensure the solution is well-mixed for a more accurate endpoint detection.

9. **Handle Reagents with Care:** Use appropriate personal protective equipment (PPE) like gloves and safety goggles, and handle all chemicals with care to avoid spills or accidents.

Gravimetric Analysis Precautions

1. **Ensure Perfect Cleanliness of Apparatus**: Clean all apparatus thoroughly before use. Fill the vessels with methylated spirits saturated with NaOH and allow them to stand for half an hour. Then, wash with water and fill with a cleaning mixture of potassium dichromate ($K_2Cr_2O_7$) and concentrated sulfuric acid (H_2SO_4), leaving it overnight. Finally, rinse thoroughly with distilled water to remove any residues, ensuring all equipment is free from contaminants.
2. **Dry the Sample Properly:** Ensure that all samples are dried to a constant weight before weighing, as moisture can affect the mass and accuracy of the analysis.
3. **Weigh Accurately:** Use an analytical balance with high precision (at least to 0.0001 grams) to weigh samples, filters, and precipitates accurately.
4. **Avoid Contamination:** Use clean, dry glassware and tools to prevent contamination that could affect the mass of the precipitate or residue.
5. **Ensure Complete Precipitation:** Follow proper procedures to ensure that precipitation is complete, as incomplete precipitation will lead to errors in the gravimetric determination.
6. **Filter and Wash Precipitates Carefully:** Use appropriate filter paper or crucibles, and wash precipitates thoroughly with distilled water to remove impurities and ensure accurate mass measurement.
7. **Dry or Ignite Precipitates to Constant Weight:** For accurate results, dry or ignite the precipitate in a drying oven or muffle furnace to a constant weight, ensuring that all volatile components are removed.
8. **Avoid Loss of Material:** Handle all samples, precipitates, and residues carefully to prevent material loss during weighing, filtering, or transferring steps.
9. **Maintain a Stable Work Environment:** Conduct gravimetric analyses in a controlled environment with minimal air currents, humidity, and temperature fluctuations, as these can affect the weight measurements.

References

Baird, C. (2017). "Environmental Chemistry" (6th ed.). W.H. Freeman.

Miller, J.C. and Miller, J.N. (2018). "Exploring Chemical Analysis" (6th ed.). W.H. Freeman.

Skoog, D.A., West, D.M., Holler, F.J., and Crouch, S.R. (2013). "Fundamentals of Analytical Chemistry" (9th ed.). Cengage Learning.

19

Study About Different Forms of Solution

The concentration of a true solution refers to the amount of solute present in a given quantity of solvent or solution. It is an important property because it determines the solution's behavior in chemical reactions, its physical properties (such as boiling and freezing points), and its utility in various applications. Concentration can be expressed in several ways, depending on the context and the precision required.

Methods to Express Concentration of a True Solution

1. Molarity (M)

- **Definition**: Molarity is the number of moles of solute dissolved in one liter (1,000 mL) of solution.
- **Formula**

$$\text{Molarity (M)} = \frac{\text{Number of moles of solute}}{\text{Volume of solution in liters}}$$

- **Units**: Moles per liter (mol/L).
- **Example**: A 1 M (1 molar) NaCl solution contains 1 mole of sodium chloride dissolved in 1 liter of water.
- **Applications**: Commonly used in laboratory settings for preparing standard solutions for titrations and other chemical analyses.

2. Molality (m)

- **Definition**: Molality is the number of moles of solute dissolved in 1 kilogram of solvent.
- **Formula**:

$$\text{Molality (m)} = \frac{\text{Number of moles of solute}}{\text{Mass of solvent in kilograms}}$$

- **Units**: Moles per kilogram (mol/kg).
- **Example**: A 1 m (1 molal) solution of glucose in water has 1 mole of glucose dissolved in 1 kg of water.
- **Applications**: Used when studying the properties of solutions, such as boiling point elevation and freezing point depression, because it is independent of temperature.

3. Normality (N)

- **Definition**: Normality is the number of gram equivalents of solute per liter of solution.
- **Formula**

$$\text{Normality (N)} = \frac{\text{Number of gram equivalents of solute}}{\text{Volume of solution in liters}}$$

- **Units**: Equivalents per liter (eq/L).
- **Example**: A 1 N solution of hydrochloric acid (HCl) contains 1 equivalent (36.5 grams) of HCl per liter of solution.
- **Applications**: Used in acid-base chemistry, redox reactions, and precipitation reactions, where the concentration of reactive species is critical.

4. Mass Percent (% w/w)

- **Definition**: Mass percent is the mass of solute divided by the total mass of the solution, multiplied by 100.
- **Formula**:

$$\text{Mass percent} = \left(\frac{\text{Mass of solute}}{\text{Mass of solution}}\right) \times 100$$

- **Units**: Percentage (%).
- **Example**: A 5% (w/w) NaCl solution contains 5 grams of NaCl in 100 grams of the solution.
- **Applications**: Widely used in industries such as pharmaceuticals, food, and chemical manufacturing to specify the concentration of solutions.

5. Volume Percent (% v/v)

- **Definition**: Volume percent is the volume of solute divided by the total volume of the solution, multiplied by 100.
- **Formula**

$$\text{Volume Percent} = \left(\frac{\text{Volume of solute}}{\text{Volume of solution}}\right) \times 100$$

- **Units**: Percentage (%).
- **Example**: A 70% (v/v) ethanol solution contains 70 mL of ethanol in 100 mL of solution.
- **Applications**: Commonly used for solutions of liquids in liquids, such as alcoholic beverages, perfumes, and cleaning agents.

6. Mass/Volume Percent (% w/v)

- **Definition**: Mass/volume percent is the mass of solute in grams per 100 milliliters of solution.
- **Formula**:

$$\text{Mass/Volume Percent} = \frac{\text{Mass of solute in grams}}{\text{Volume of solution in mililiters}} \times 100$$

- **Units**: Percentage (%).
- **Example**: A 5% (w/v) glucose solution contains 5 grams of glucose in 100 mL of solution.
- **Applications**: Often used in medical and biological contexts, such as the preparation of intravenous (IV) fluids.

7. Mole Fraction (χ)

- **Definition**: Mole fraction is the ratio of the number of moles of solute to the total number of moles of all components in the solution.
- **Formula**:

$$\text{Mole Fraction of Solute } (\chi) = \frac{\text{Number of moles of solute}}{\text{Total number of moles of solute and solvent}}$$

- **Units**: Dimensionless (no units).
- **Example**: In a solution with 1 mole of ethanol and 4 moles of water, the mole fraction of ethanol is 1/ (1+4) = 0.2.
- **Applications**: Used in colligative property calculations, such as vapor pressure lowering and osmotic pressure.

8. Parts Per Million (ppm) and Parts Per Billion (PPB)

- **Definition**:
- **ppm**: Number of parts of solute per million parts of solution.
- **ppb**: Number of parts of solute per billion parts of solution.
- **Formula**

$$\text{ppm} = \left(\frac{\text{Mass of solute}}{\text{Mass of solution}}\right) \times 10^6$$

$$\text{ppb} = \left(\frac{\text{Mass of solute}}{\text{Mass of solution}}\right) \times 10^9$$

- **Units**: ppm or ppb.
- **Example**: A solution with 1 mg of solute in 1 liter of water is 1 ppm.
- **Applications**: Used in environmental science, chemistry, and toxicology to measure low concentrations of pollutants, contaminants, and trace elements.

9. Formality (F)

- **Definition**: Formality is the number of formula units of solute per liter of solution. It is similar to molarity, but it is used when the solute does not completely dissociate into ions.
- **Formula**

$$\text{Formality (F)} = \frac{\text{Number of gram formula units of solute}}{\text{Volume of solution in liters}}$$

- **Units**: Formula units per liter.
- **Example**: A 1 F solution of NaCl contains 1 gram formula unit of NaCl per liter of solution.

- **Applications**: Used in chemistry when dealing with compounds that do not dissociate completely in solution.

References

Atkins, P., & de Paula, J. (2014). *Physical Chemistry*. Oxford University Press.

Brown, T.L., LeMay, H.E., Bursten, B.E., & Murphy, C.J. (2017). *Chemistry: The Central Science*. Pearson.

Greenwood, N. N., & Earnshaw, A. (1997). *Chemistry of the Elements*. Butterworth-Heinemann.

Silberberg, M. S. (2015). *Chemistry: The Molecular Nature of Matter and Change*. McGraw-Hill Education.

Plates

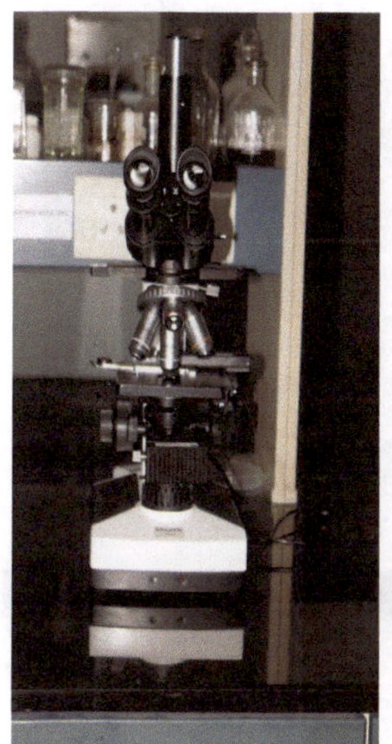

Binocular Research Microscope

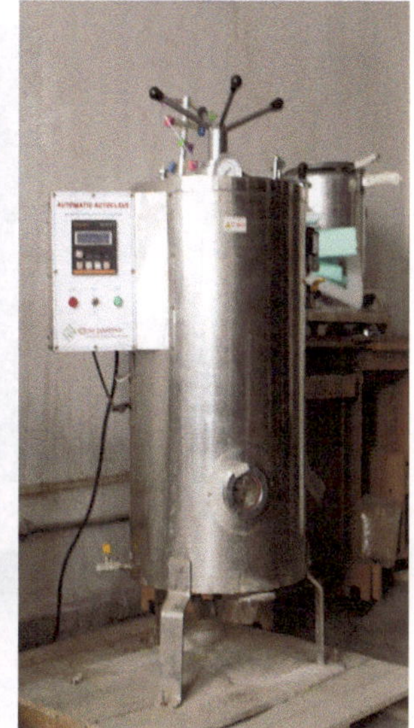

Autoclave

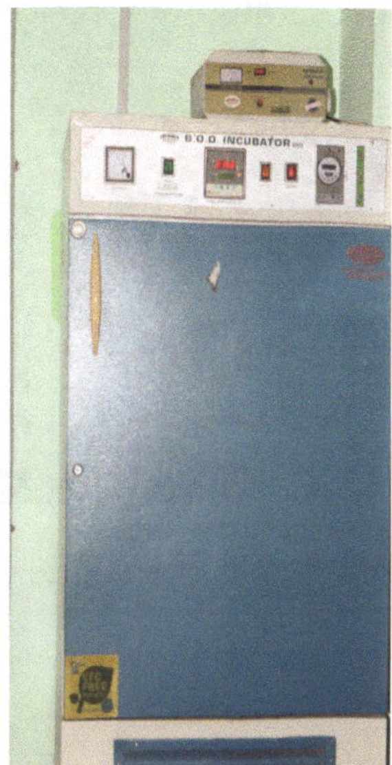

BOD Incubator

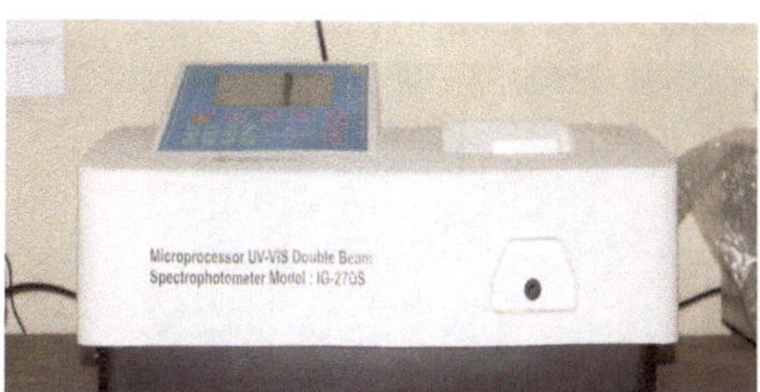

Microprocessor UV-VIS Double Beam Spectrophotometer

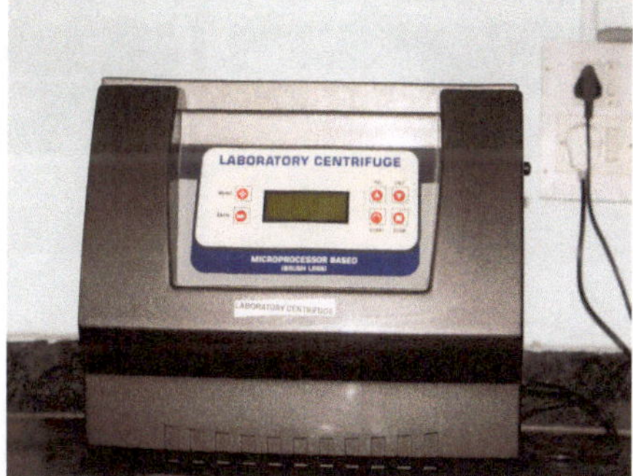

Centrifuge

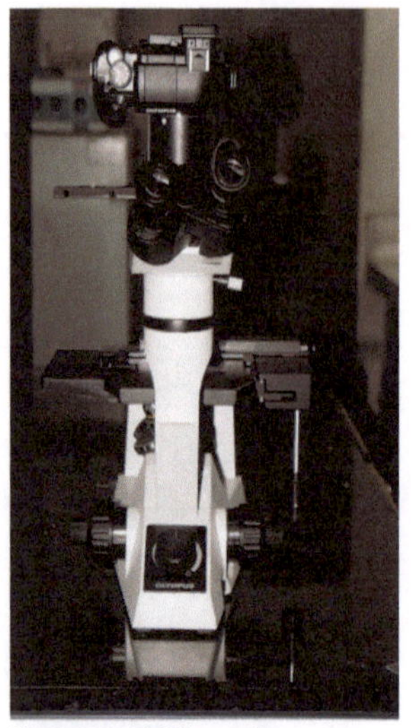
Compound Binocular Microscope

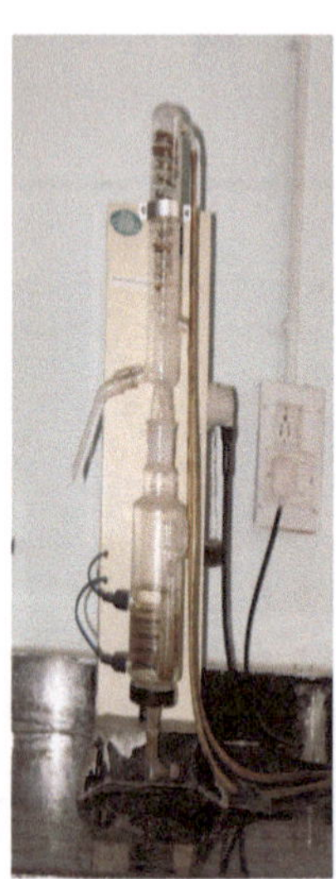
Double Distiller

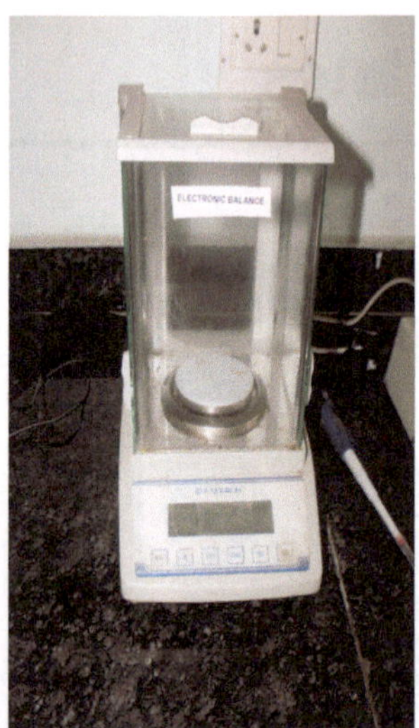
Electronic Balance

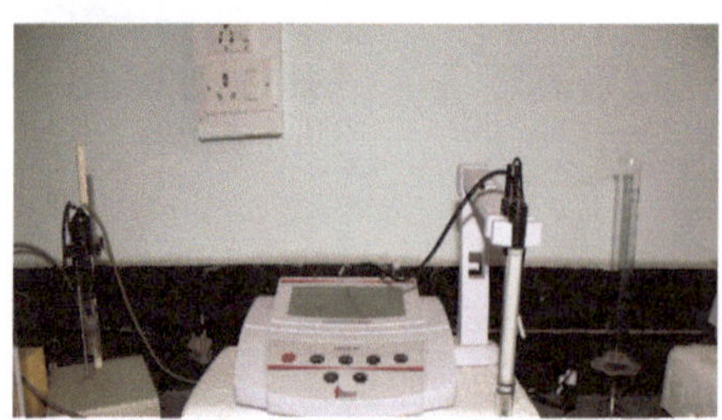
Conductivity Meter

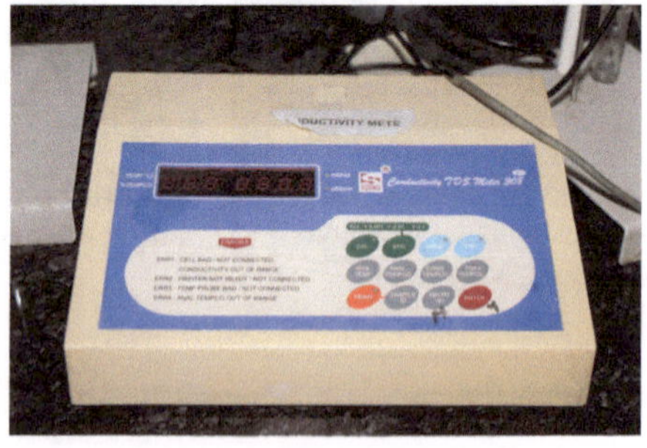
Conductivity TDS Meter

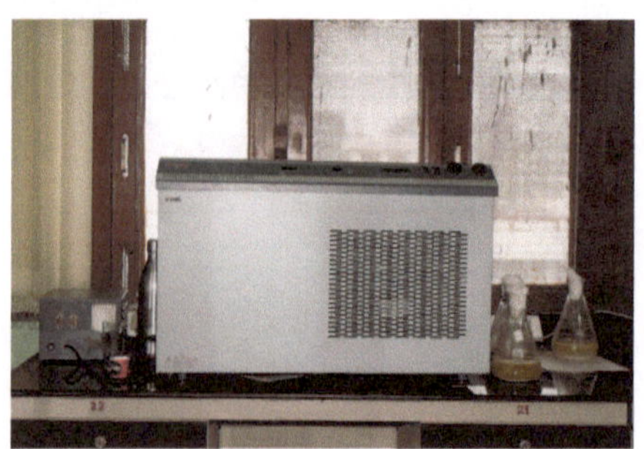
Cooling Centrifuge

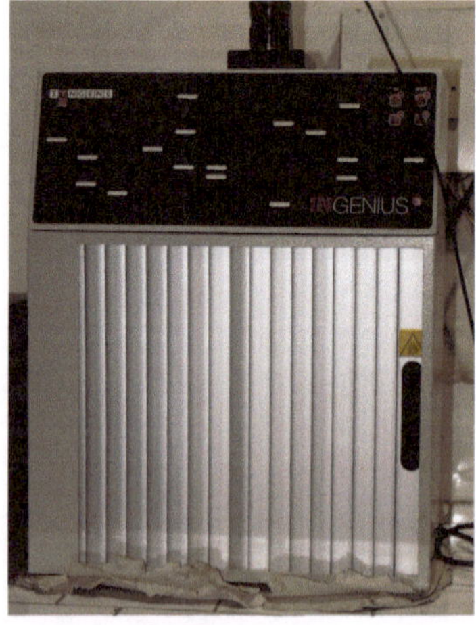

Gel Documentation

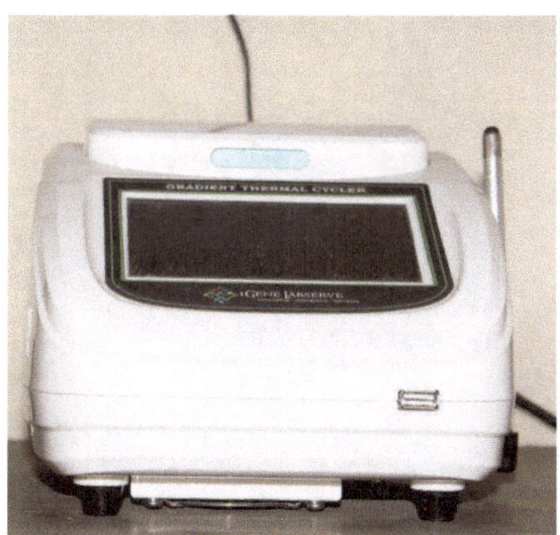

Gradient Thermal Cycler

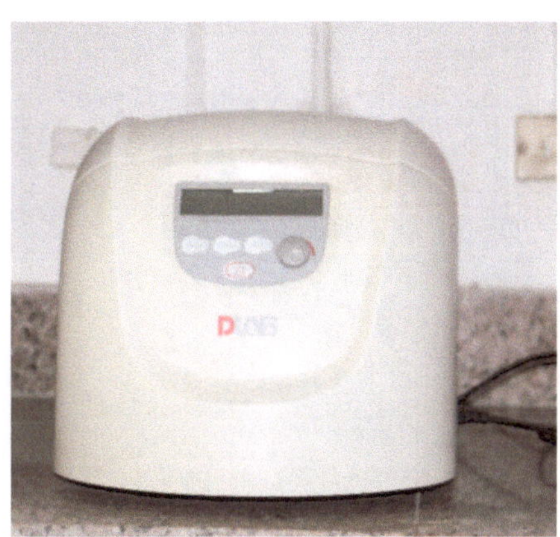

High Speed Micro Centrifuge

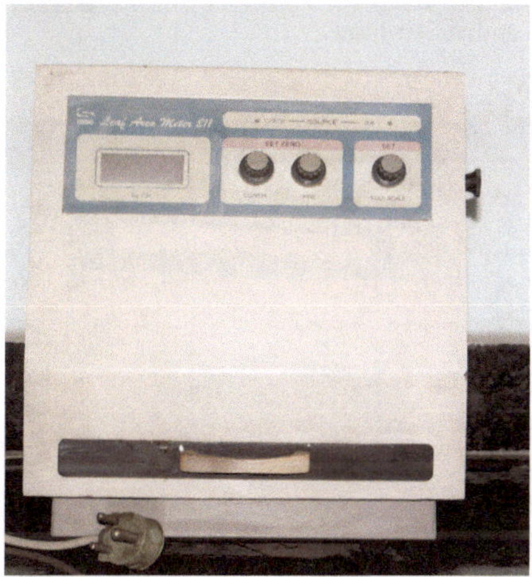

Leaf Area Meter

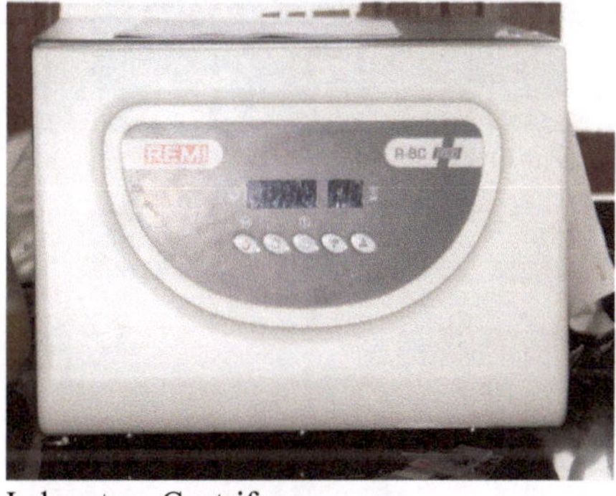

Laboratory Centrifuge

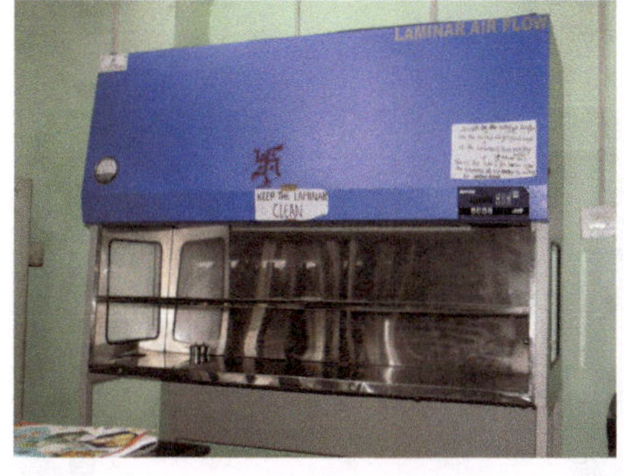

Laminar Air Flow

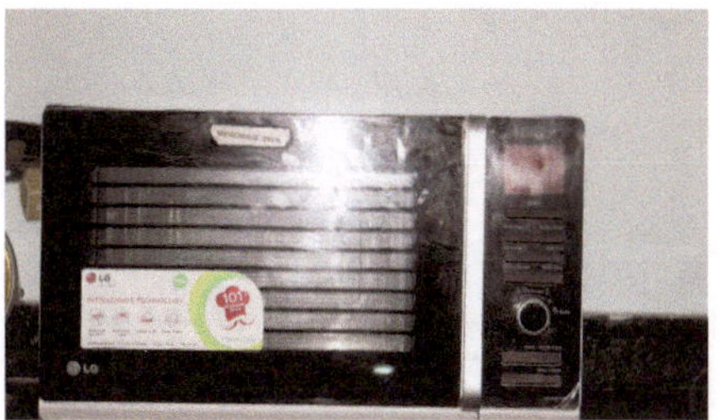

Microoven

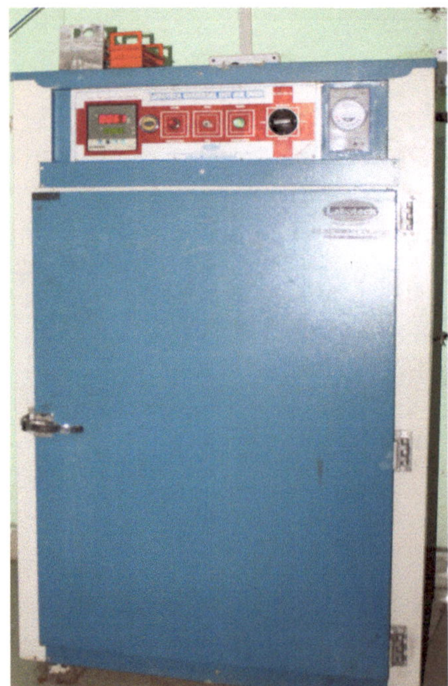

Hot Air Oven

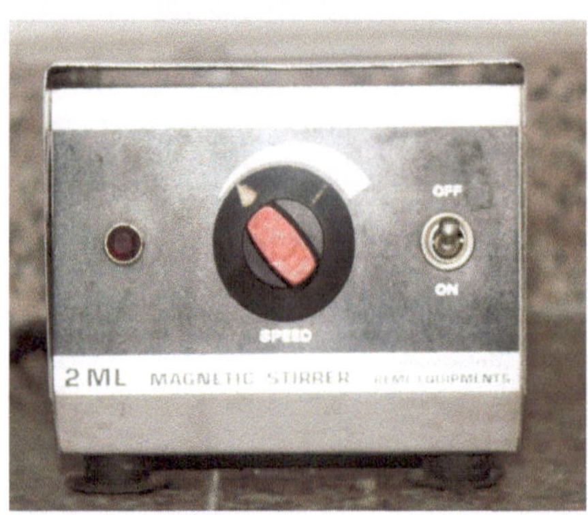

Magnetic Stirrer

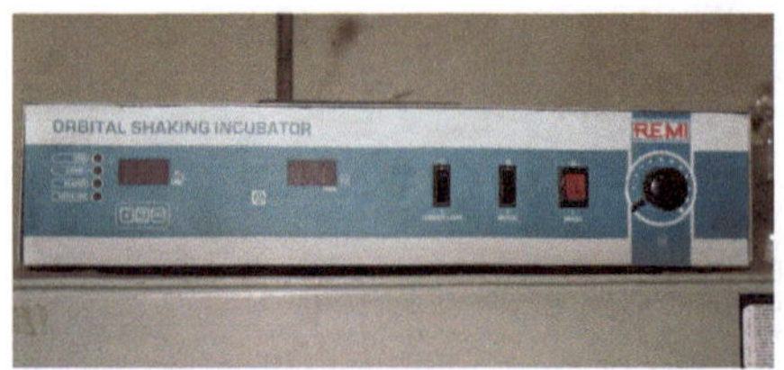

Orbital Shaking Incubator

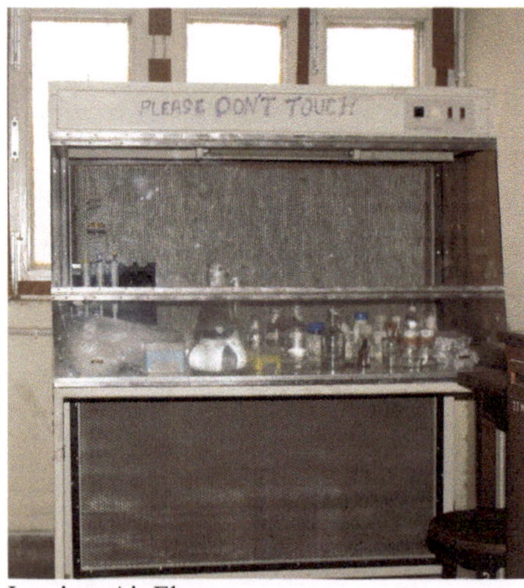

Laminar Air Flow

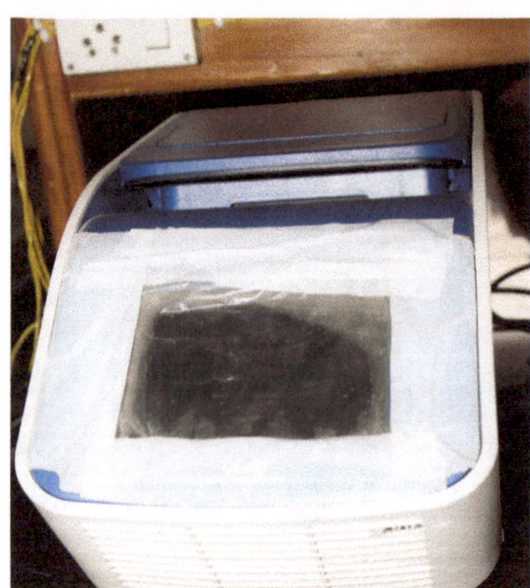

thermo-cycler

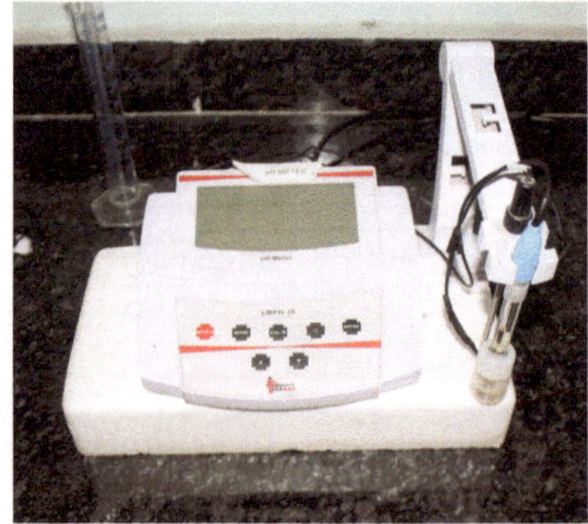

pH Meter

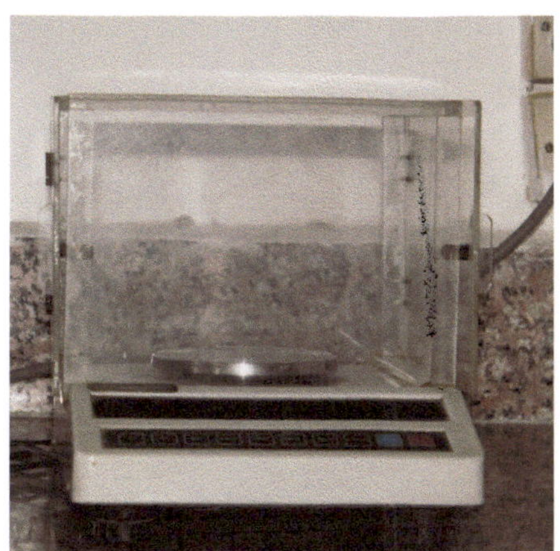
weighing balance

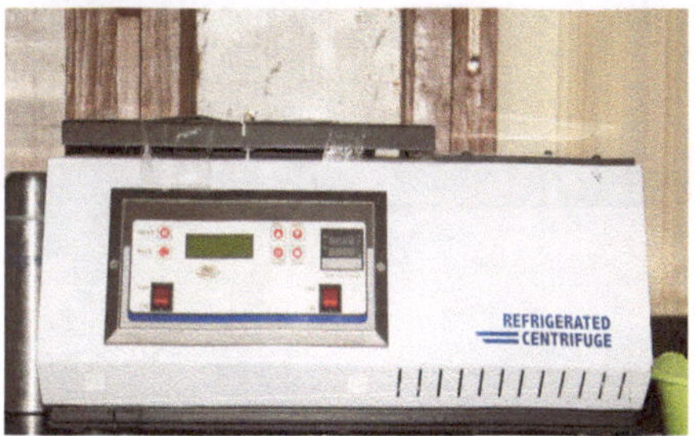

Refrigerated Centrifuge

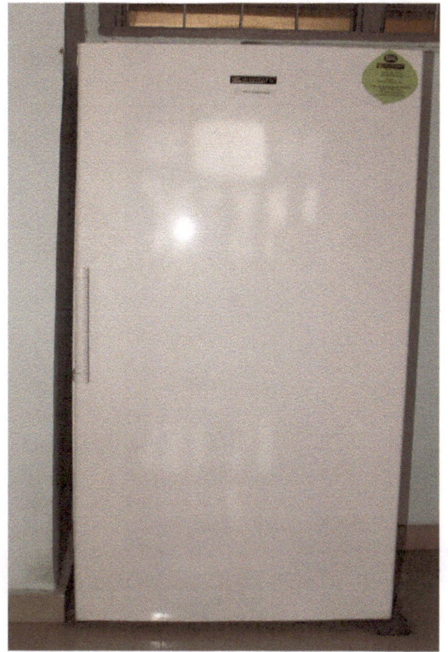
Refrigerator

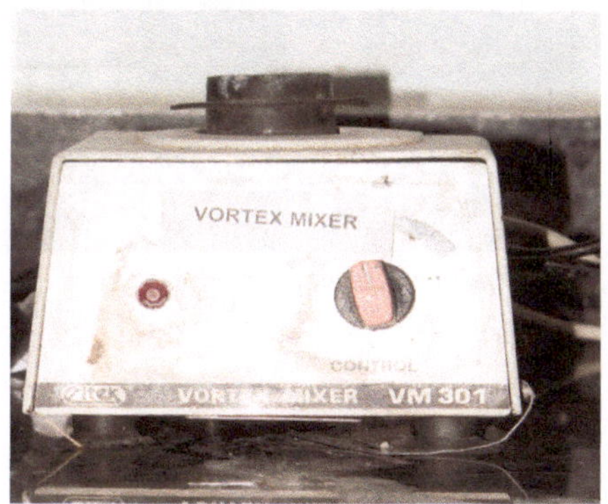

Vortex Mixer

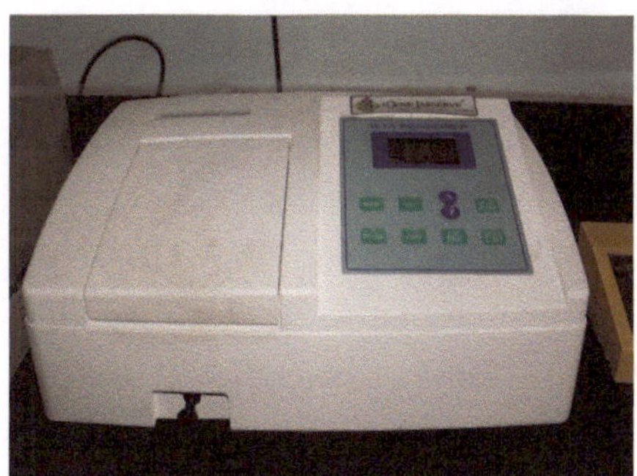
Spectrophotometer

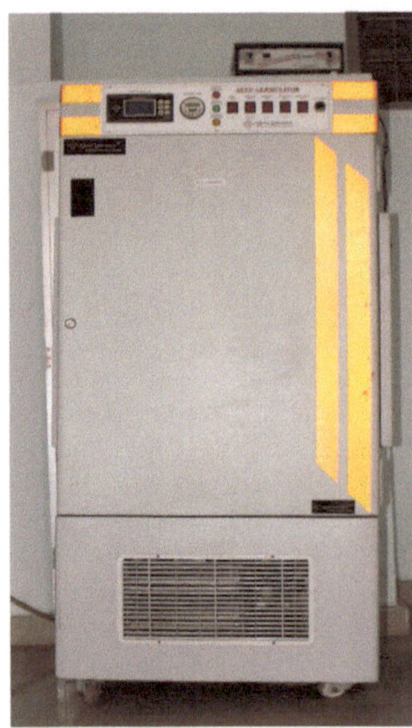

Seed Germinator

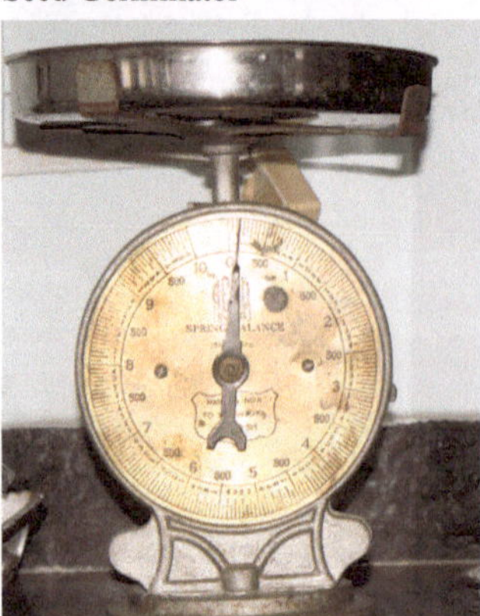

Spring Balance

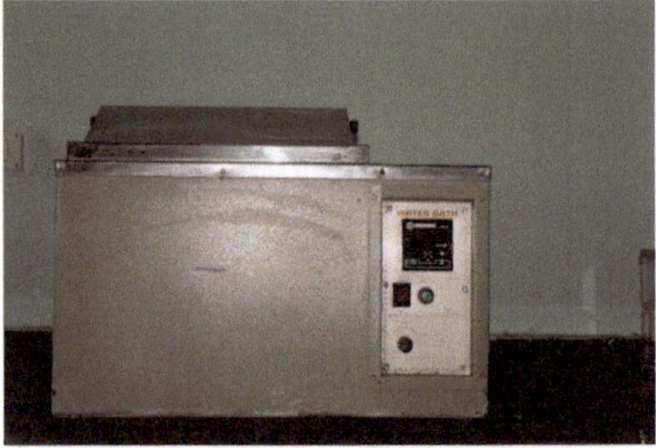

Water Bath

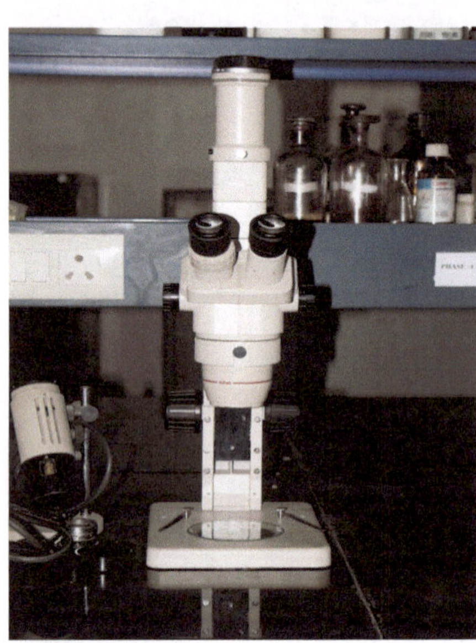

Stereo Zoom Microscope

Index

A
Acid: 5, 6, 7, 8, 9, 11, 14, 26, 27, 28, 29, 30, 33, 34, 35, 36, 39, 40, 41, 47, 48, 51, 52, 53, 68, 71, 72, 73, 74, 75, 77, 78, 82
Agriculture: 5
Agronomy: 2, 4, 6, 8, 10, 12, 14, 16, 18, 20, 22, 26, 28, 30, 34, 36, 40, 42, 44, 48, 52, 53, 56, 60, 62, 64, 68, 70, 72, 74, 76, 78, 82, 84
Ammonium: 2, 3, 14, 15, 16, 27, 28, 35, 51, 52, 53

B
Base: 3, 4, 21, 22, 27, 28, 30, 35, 41, 45, 55, 56, 62, 68, 71, 72, 73, 77, 82
Beneficial:
Buffer: 48, 71, 72, 73, 74, 75, 76

C
Chlorine: 1, 2, 3, 11, 12, 14, 33
Chlorophyll: 5, 7, 8, 9, 27, 55, 56, 57, 62, 65
Deficiency:

F
Functional: 1, 2

N
Nitrogen: 2, 3, 5, 6, 8, 9, 11, 14, 17, 25, 26, 27, 28, 29, 30, 31
Nutrition: 1, 7, 13

P
Physiological: 5, 6, 7, 9, 11, 17, 18
Physiology: 2, 4, 6, 8, 10, 11, 12, 14, 16, 18, 20, 22, 26, 28, 30, 34, 36, 40, 42, 44, 48, 52, 56, 57, 60, 62, 63, 64, 65, 68, 70, 72, 74, 76, 78, 82, 84
Sample: 14, 19, 20, 21, 22, 23, 25, 26, 27, 28, 29, 30, 31, 33, 34, 36, 37, 39, 40, 41, 43, 44, 45, 47, 48, 51, 53, 55, 56, 57, 59, 60, 61, 63, 64, 65, 78
Sodium: 2, 3, 14, 20, 28, 30, 33, 43, 72, 73, 74, 75, 76, 81

T
Titration: 27, 28, 29, 30, 41, 51, 52, 53, 77, 81
Toxicity: 5, 6, 7, 8, 9, 10, 11, 12, 43